Vedda Blood Sugar Remedy

Michael Dempsey

Copyright © 2017 Michael Dempsey

All rights reserved.

ISBN: 9781549845314

Readers are advised to consult with their physician or another professional practitioner before implementing any suggestions that follow. This book is not intended to take the place of sound professional advice, medical or otherwise. Neither the author nor the publisher assumes any liability for possible adverse consequences as a result of the information contained herein.

CONTENTS

1	INTRODUCTION	1
2	DIABETES DOES NOT DEFINE YOU	5
3	THE TROUBLE WITH CONVENTIONAL MEDICATIONS	18
4	THE NASTY TRUTH ABOUT SUGAR	23
5	THE REAL WAY TO DROP THE EXCESS WEIGHT	37
6	WISDOM OF THE VEDDA	48
7	THE SECRET INGREDIENTS OF THE VEDDA THAT ELIMINATE DIABETES	56
8	VEDDA LIFESTYLE FACTORS	72
9	THE FULL BODY DETOX	85
10	YOUR DIABETES - FREE FUTURE	124

Copyright: Published in the United States by Michael Dempsey/ © Michael Dempsey

All rights reserved. No part of this publication may be reproduced, stored in retrieval system, copied in any form or by any means, electronic, mechanical, photocopying, recording or otherwise transmitted without written permission from the publisher. Please do not participate in or encourage piracy of this material in any way. You must not circulate this book in any format. Brian Wilds does not control or direct users' actions and is not responsible for the information or content shared, harm and/or actions of the book readers. In accordance with the U.S. Copyright Act of 1976, the scanning, uploading and electronic sharing of any part of this book without the permission of the publisher constitute unlawful piracy and theft of the author's intellectual prope

I. INTRODUCTION

What was your first reaction when you learned that you had diabetes? Did you jump online and Google the word, only to be confronted with thousands of alarming results – and no clear answers?

That's what 99.7 percent of people who have just been hit with the bad news do – they seek out the latest, most technological answer available.

If you're like most people, you no doubt, peppered Google with the obvious questions:

What is diabetes? What is the treatment? How will diabetes affect me?

Google no doubt happily obliged by spitting out endless information for you to wade through. But it may not have taken you long to notice that the information

presented was full of contradictions, errors, and downright fabrications. Well, it's time to thank the internet for its well-meaning advice and go get a second opinion. Your health depends on it.

As you are about to discover, the real solution to diabetes lies, not in the latest technology, but in the wisdom of the ancients – specifically the dietary habits of a small native group of inhabitants based in the jungles of Sri Lanka.

Before you can get better answers, however, you need to start asking better questions. Questions that will give you individual answers that relate to your situation. Answers that will fit your lifestyle and that are practical, realistic, and workable for you.

- Why is this happening to me now?
- What can I do, without pumping my body full of drugs, to heal my affected organs?
- What lifestyle factors will help me to recover my health?
- What is wrong with my current treatment and what can I do about it?
- How can I stay on top of my diabetes without breaking the bank?

Those are the very questions I asked when my family's life was thrown into turmoil. My wife, Robyn, nearly died of a diabetic heart attack. Once I'd processed the shock of it, I ran to Google, too.

Little did I realize that the solution that I – and every person who is affected by diabetes – needed came from the brain of a ninety-one-year-old forest dwelling native of Sri Lanka who'd never turned on a computer in his life!

That wisdom comes from the Vedda people of the jungles of Sri Lanka – a people who have NEVER had a documented case of diabetes.

I put my complete trust – and my wife's life – in the hands of this old man. With what result?

In less than a month, my wife Rachel slashed her blood sugar readings from a potentially fatal 605 milligrams per deciliter, all the way down to a safe and stable 120 in the space of just thirty-three days, and completely reversed her diabetes.

She also eradicated her paralysis, reversed her nerve damage, lowered her blood pressure and cholesterol, and shed a whopping thirty-five pounds at the same time.

The book that you are now reading details everything that allowed Rachel to achieve those amazing results.

You can think of this protocol as the Vedda Diet 2.0. This is a powerful and effective diabetes-reversing program that everyone suffering from the disease should take to heart.

Inside the guide, you will discover everything you need to know about the Vedda people, their diet, and their lifestyle, which has made them virtually immune to diabetes.

You will discover why today's diabetes medications can't, won't, and never will cure you of this disease, but will actually make your symptoms worse.

I'll show you the clinical studies which inspired this treatment program and demonstrate how you can prevent, stop, and reverse diabetes is by eating a small selection of very simple foods.

But that's not even the best part.

As well as the main ingredients list, the book also includes my most powerful and easy- to-prepare Blood Sugar Lowering Recipes. The recipes are complete with the exact ingredients, amounts, and combinations used in our most successful trials.

Each recipe also includes a full shopping list and has been specifically designed to remove all of the hard work from your daily meal planning, so you can gain control over your blood sugar levels, defeat your diabetes, and transform your health and waistline with the minimum of fuss.

And finally, the pièce de résistance: my 30-Day Blood Sugar Protocol, where you will find our most ruthlessly effective 30- day meal plan for reversing your diabetes permanently.

Are you ready to start watching your blood sugar readings fall day after day until your doctor gives you the thumbs up and tells you that you no longer need to take medication anymore?

How about seeing the weight start falling off so that you can fit into the jeans you haven't worn in years? If this sounds appealing, keep reading and we'll begin.

II. DIABETES DOES NOT DEFINE YOU

Diabetes Does Not Define You

Do you remember your emotional state when you first found out that you had diabetes? Did it seem that your life suddenly became much more constricted? Amid the anxiety, the confusion, the fear and the anger did you feel that many of your opportunities for fulfilment were slipping away? Maybe you wanted to be an athlete like the mighty heavy-weight champ Joe Frazier. Or a brilliant author like Ernest Hemingway. Your ambition may have been to entertain others like Tom Hanks or Halle Berry. Or, was it to be a musical entrepreneur like Randy Jackson?

All of those people are diabetes sufferers – and all of them enjoy incredibly fulfilling lives. So can you. Diabetes doesn't define those celebrities. You may even be surprised to learn that they are or were diabetics. It hasn't ruined their health and it hasn't made them give up on their dreams. They have learned how to control their diabetes and gone on to live full, exciting lives.

You can do the same.

So, Just What Is Diabetes Anyway?

Remember the guy who said, "Knowledge is Power?"

No, neither do we – but, whoever he was, he was on to something. By learning about this disease you'll be able to understand what in your body is not going right. You'll then be in a position to make adjustments.

When someone has diabetes, it means that they have too much glucose in their blood. Glucose is the body's main source of energy. We turn glucose from the food we eat into energy. Our bodies need energy to grow and repair themselves, and we need energy for everything we do. We all take in energy from many different foods, including pasta, bread, and potatoes. As our bodies digest this food it is broken down into glucose. We all need glucose because our bodies turn it into energy.

The buildup of glucose in the bloodstream leads to the release of extra insulin, for the purpose of directing the glucose into our cells.

The glucose is absorbed by the cells and the level of glucose in the blood drops. Our hunger hormones then kick in to restock our energy levels. At the same time, the liver releases some stored glucose while, simultaneously, signaling the pancreas to release less insulin. In this way, the various parts of the body work together to achieve a state of homeostasis, or balance.

In people who have diabetes, the body is unable to turn glucose into energy. Instead of being used up, the glucose builds up in their blood. It also means that they are unable to get the energy they need from the food they eat. This can make them feel weak and tired.

Diabetics are unable to make the best use of a chemical called insulin.

The body makes insulin in a gland called the pancreas, which lies across the back of the stomach. Insulin is needed to use the sugar in the blood for energy. It also controls the level of glucose in the blood.

There are two main types of diabetes. Type-1 diabetes is more common in children.

When they are very young, their pancreas stops making insulin. No one really knows why this happens. Without any insulin, they cannot make energy. Instead, all the sugar in their food stays in their blood or is passed out of the body in their urine.

Type-2 diabetes tends to start in older people and is more common than Type 1. With Type-2 diabetes, the pancreas can still make insulin but the rest of the body can't use it properly. The result is the same as with Type-1 diabetes – there is too much glucose in the blood. This excess glucose makes its way to the various parts of your body, where it is stored and clogs up the function of those body areas. Meanwhile, the cells are starving for glucose but can't get it. As a result, the person feels, weak, lethargic, and generally horrible.

A related condition is known as insulin resistance. A person who has insulin resistance produces a normal amount of insulin from the pancreas but the cells of the body are unable to use the insulin effectively.

Diabetes and your Kidneys

The kidneys are the main organ of the body that are affected by diabetes. You have two kidneys and, oddly enough, they are shaped like kidney beans. They are locat- ed just above the waist in the back of the abdomen. About 25 percent of the blood pumped by your heart goes to your kid- neys. To receive all of this blood, the kidneys contain a whole lot of extremely fine blood vessels. But diabetes causes these vessels to thicken. It also causes damage to them.

Over time the vessels may begin to leak. This can cause essential nutrients, like proteins, to be released into the urine. In addition, the removal of waste products from the body may be impaired, leading to major health problems and the condition known as diabetic kidney disease.

More than two thousandyearsago, diabetes was known around the Roman Empire as the "disease of the kidneys." Over the centuries, however, the major role played by the kidneys was downplayed. Today, we appreciate the vital role that the kidneys play in maintaining glucose homeostasis. They do this by filtering, reabsorbing, and excreting glucose. When this process is functioning properly, we are in a state of glucose balance. When it is not, we will end up either hyperglycemic (too much blood glucose) or hypoglycemic (not enough blood glucose).

What Causes Diabetes?

There's a lot of media attention lately directed to the lifestyle factors that cause diabetes. But there are also unavoidable risk factors that contribute to the condition. These are the things that you have no control over and, therefore, are unable to change. Here are the main unavoidable risk factors:

Age – as we age the regenerative capacity of the pancreas slows down and its ability to make insulin declines. Despite the fact that an alarming number of people under twenty-five are developing the condition, most people who are diagnosed with Type- 2 diabetes are aged between fifty-five and sixty.

- Family History – one in every three people with Type-2 diabetes has a close family member who also has the condition.
- Race – People of certain ethnic origins, such as African Americans,
- Hispanics, American Indians and Asian- Americans, are more likely to develop Type-2 diabetes.
- Pre-existing health conditions – High blood pressure, metabolic syndrome, impaired glucose tolerance along with heart disease, and stroke all put you at higher risk of getting diabetes.
- Viruses – Infections such as mumps, rubella, adenovirus, cytomegalovirus, and coxsackievirus B can lead to the onset of Type-2 diabetes
- Bottle feeding – A number of recent studies have linked formula feeding with cow's milk to Type-2 diabetes. Breastfeeding is highly recommended, as is supplementing with vitamin D.
- Liver or pancreatic disease – Any condition that impairs the ability of the pancreas and liver to do their job is going to make you more likely to become diabetic. There are some vital other factors that are major contributors to type-2 diabetes. These ones come under the category of lifestyle factors – they are things that we can control and make choices around.

Here are the main avoidable risk factors:

- Obesity - The fat cells that are located in the abdomen are responsible for the secretion of hormones, the regulators of all of our bodily functions. When we have too many fat cells located around the abdominal regions, we tend to secrete more hormones and chemicals that slow down our metabolisms. And the result of that is likely to be an inefficient insulin metabolism process. This hormone-induced insulin resistance is directly related to high blood pressure, abnormal blood fats, and Type-2 Diabetes.

- Lack of Exercise – Exercise not only burns calories, it offsets insulin. Exercise increases the uptake of glucose, both during and after exercise, meaning less work for insulin and other medications.
- Diet – a diet that is high in sugar, saturated fat, cholesterol, and trans fats increases the work of the pancreas and can lead to obesity.
- Alcohol – too much alcohol consumption suppresses the production of glucose by the liver. It also can permanently damage the pancreas.
- Smoking – toxins contained in cigarette smoke stress the surface of blood vessels and increase your blood pressure and cholesterol levels. As a result, smoking will make you 70 percent more likely to become diabetic.

Red Flag Organs

The human body is a complementary organism composed of an amazingly complex system of cells. Its fifteen bodily systems are inter-related. If we incur weakness in one system, that weakness will be reflected in another system. In essence, wewillonlybe as healthyas the unhealthiest system in our body. Within our bodies there are certain key organs that we rely upon for a host of functions that weave through a number of bodily systems. Three of the most important are the liver, the pancreas, and the kidneys. If their optimal functioning is compromised, we are increasing our likelihood of developing diabetes

The Liver

One of the key functions of the liver is to store blood sugars or glucose. The liver also regulates the circulating blood sugars in the body, keeping them at optimum levels. But the liver doesn't just store glucose. It also has the ability to manufacture it. The signals to either store or to manufacture glucose come from chemical messengers known as hormones. The two key hormones relating to blood sugar are insulin and glucagon.

The food you eat goes into the stomach. The stomach breaks down the food and it gets absorbed in the body as blood sugar, which floats around in your bloodstream. When we eat, insulin is secreted by specialized cells in the pancreas. At the same time, glucagon is suppressed. Insulin enables glucose to enter muscle and fat cells, where it is used as energy and stored for future use in the form of glycogen.

When the body is in need of energy, such as when you are undergoing a fast, the liver has the ability to convert stored glucose into energy for the body to use. The body also has a glycogen sparing response when your body's glycogen stores get too low. It will horde the sugar and direct it to the brain, the kidneys, and the red blood cells.

The liver doesn't just rely upon stored blood sugars to create energy. By means of a process known as "gluconeogenesis" it can convert proteins and fats into energy for the body to use. In response to lowered insulin levels, the body will turn to stored fat as its preferred energy source in a process known as ketogenesis.

The liver is meant to take a portion of that blood sugar and store it as energy. A clogged liver, however, cannot store blood sugar as effectively. As a result, you'll have more blood sugars floating around in your system.

In order to get the blood sugars out, the pancreas pumps out insulin. Over time this creates a cycle effect where the person becomes resistant to their own insulin. This creates insulin resistance. This is essentially what type 2 diabetes is, the inability of the body to use its own insulin properly.

By clearing up the liver and getting it working properly, you'll be able to store excess blood sugars and your blood sugar will start to drop.

With the liver being so vital in the glucose equation, it's clear to see that a less than optimally functioning liver can be a contributor to Type 2 diabetes. Recent studies indicate that people who suffer from Hepatitis C are more likely to develop diabetes than non sufferers.

It is ironic to note, however, that a popular treatment for Hepatitis B and C can actually contribute to the development of Type 2 diabetes. Interferon therapy utilizes weekly injections to control Hepatitis. One of the possible side effects is hyperglycemia which can, in turn, trigger Type 2 diabetes. In addition, Interferon injections can contribute to Type 1 diabetes as a result of Interferon's ability to develop insulin auto- antibodies.

Diabetes makes a person twice as likely to develop both pancreatic and liver cancer. Acute liver failure, in which damaged cells are unable to be replaced by healthy cells, is a fatal condition. During acute liver failure, the organ is unable to adequately store glucose, resulting in enhanced insulin levels and low glucose levels. Organ transplants, especially a liver transplant, can make people more susceptible to diabetes. One study indicated that 40 percent of liver transplant patients developed diabetes within three years of their procedure.

Hemochromatosis is a disease that damages the pancreas, in addition to the liver, the heart, joints, and the nervous system. It results from the excessive absorption of iron into the blood, which, in turn, delivers an abnormal amount of iron to the liver and heart. Unless treated it can lead to liver disease, cirrhosis, and diabetes.

The Unwell Pancreas

Your pancreas sits below your stomach. Its two key functions are to produce digestive enzymes that break down food and to produce and secrete insulin into the bloodstream. Wherever insulin travels in your body, it opens up the cells so that glucose can enter them. This allows the cells to access the energy they need to function. If your pancreas is unwell and can't produce insulin as the body needs it, you will be either hypoglycemic with unhealthy low levels of blood glucose or hyperglycemic with far too much blood glucose circulating around your body.

The main afflictions affecting the pancreas are:

- **Pancreatic Exocrine Syndromes**: A number of pancreatic disorders that are commonly caused by such lifestyle factors as smoking, alcohol abuse, and unhealthy dietary choices come under this umbrella, including:
- **Pancreatitis** – inflammation where the digestive enzymes start digesting the pancreas itself
- **Cystic Fibrosis** – pancreatic tubes are blocked by a thick, sticky mucus
- **Pancreatic cancer** – symptoms include yellowing of skin, abdominal pain, weight loss and fatigue.
- **Pancreatic Viruses**: The following viruses, which directly affect the pancreas, increase the risk of diabetes.

This has been seen to be as a result of anti-islet antibodies that cause damage to the beta cells which produce insulin:

1. Congenital Rubella Syndrome

2. Cytomegalovirus

RED FLAG ALERT
Type 2 Diabetes: The New Children's Epidemic

There's a new epidemic sweeping the globe and it is targeting our children. Type 2 diabetes used to be an adults-only condition. In fact, it used to be called adult- onset diabetes.

But, no more.

The number of children with type 2 diabetes has skyrocketed over the past twenty years. That's why it has been referred to by such prestigious publications as Diabetes Care as an emerging epidemic.

What Causes Type 2 Diabetes in Children?

Diabetes is often referred to as a lifestyle disease. That is because the main factors that lead to diabetes can be controlled.

These are the three key causes of type 2 diabetes among children:

- Obesity – The fat cells that are located in the abdomen are responsible for the secretion of hormones, the regulators of all of our bodily functions. When we have too many fat cells located around the abdominal region, we tend to secrete more hormones and chemicals that slow down our metabolism. And the result of that is likely to be an inefficient insulin metabolism process. This hormone-induced insulin resistance is directly related to high blood pressure, abnormal blood fats, and type 2 diabetes.
- Lack of Exercise – Exercise not only burns calories, it offsets insulin. Exercise increases the uptake of glucose, both during and after exercise, meaning less work for insulin and other medications.

- Diet — a diet that is high in sugar, saturated fat, cholesterol and trans fats increases the work of the pancreas and can lead to obesity.

Making the Change

The good news about type 2 diabetes is that change is possible. It is never too early or too late to start children on a course of exercise and nutrition that will steer them away from diabetes.

Here's how:

Limit Their Intake of Sugary Foods and Beverages

While sugar is in most food products, three favorites among children are soft drinks, fruit juices, and energy drinks.

Here is why you must STOP giving these drinks to your child today.

Energy drinks, fruit juices, and sodas attack a child's body on two fronts as the combined effects of glucose and fructose play havoc with the system. Blood sugar levels will get an immediate spike from the glucose. In response to this, the pancreas will elevate its insulin manufacture.

The fructose in the drink will fast track it to the liver, where it is converted into fat, with the byproducts of triglycerides and uric acid. Meanwhile, the excess amount of insulin in the system will stimulate your child's appetite.

Now, remember that all of this has resulted from a liquid — the child hasn't eaten anything. Yet, the child now has a craving to do just that. When he or she reaches for something sweet, the whole destructive process is replicated. That's why energy drinks, sodas, and fruit juices don't belong in your child's life.

Make the smarter choice for your child and offer natural fruits and vegetables, which come ready packed with vitamins, minerals, amino acids, and anti-oxidants.

Get Regular Exercise

Too much time in front of a screen is a major contributor to childhood diabetes. As a parent, you have the obligation to ensure that your child turns off technology and gets out in the fresh air. Children need to move their bodies vigorously every day.

Here are five tips to get your child active:

- Exercise and play sports with your child. Get bicycles and ride together. Go to a park on the weekends and play soccer or basketball. Go for walks in the woods. Get out and enjoy nature with your child.
- Place a limit on screen time.
- Give your child chores to do around the home. Get him or her vacuum cleaning, taking out the garbage, and mowing the lawn.
- Be a model of health and fitness to your children. Let them see you taking your health seriously by eating and drinking wisely and exercising.
- Encourage your children to get actively involved in sporting opportunities at school. Encourage them to join a team, or try out for a competitive sport.

Conclusion

There is no doubt that type 2 diabetes is running rampant among our children. But that doesn't mean that we have to stand by idly and watch them suffer. It is up to us, the parents, to do something about it. Steering our children toward a lifestyle of regular exercise and sensible eating habits could well be the most precious gift we ever give them.

III. THE TROUBLE WITH CONVENTIONAL MEDICATIONS

Some medications that patients receive for initialtreatment oftype 2 diabetescancause harmful side effects without addressing the underlying causes of diabetes. When patients have difficulty changing their dietary habits or lifestyles, doctors often resort to prescription medication.

The basic premise behind diabetic drugs is that they will lower blood sugar levels. However, this completely misses the point. You see, type 2 diabetes is not a blood sugar disease. It is a lifestyle disease. Type 2 diabetics do not necessarily need drugs – they need to change their lifestyles.

In a recent meta-analysis study, thirty- three thousand diabetics were analyzed to see how doctor-prescribed medications affected them long term. It was shown that the treatments were not only ineffective, they were downright dangerous. Here's what the researchers concluded.

"The overall results of this meta-analysis do not show a benefit of intensive glucose- lowering treatment on all-cause mortality or cardiovascular death. A 19 percent increase in all-cause mortality and a 43 percent increase in cardiovascular mortality cannot be excluded."

The most popular diabetic drug in the world is Metformin. It is the only drug that has been proven to decrease the chance of heart attack. It is an oral diabetes medicine that helps control blood sugar levels and is designed for type 2 diabetics.

Metformin was discovered in 1922 as an anti-diabetic drug. It came on the market at the same time that scientists were able to make synthetic insulin. It was first brought to Europe in 1958 and to Canada in 1992. It arrived in the USA in 1995.

The Metformin molecule is derived from a French lilac flower, which has been prescribed for hundreds of years to treat problems associated with excess sugar in the urine. Metformin works on the liver's production of glucose.

People take Metformin because they get diagnosed with high blood sugar. A complication associated with high blood sugar is the risk of cardiovascular disease. However, what many patients don't realize is that Metformin can actually make them worse.

The list of dangers associated with Metformin is daunting. They include

- Dizziness
- Digestive problems
- Hormonal disruption
- Sinus Infection

When you deplete the body's Vitamin B12 levels, you are at a heightened risk of cardiovascular disease. A 2010 study showed the Metformin drastically reduces your B12 levels.

That's a major problem.

Vitamin B12 deficiency can make you prone to heart attacks and other cardiovascular problems.

Metformin also lowers your folate levels. This leads to impaired immune function, chronic low energy, poor digestion, anemia, mood swings, and pale skin.

Another commonly prescribed drug is Avandia. This drug came out in 1999. A 2007 study revealed just how dangerous it was. Published in the New England Journal of Medicine, it linked the use of Avandia to a 43-percent increase in heart attack risk and a 64-percent jump in the risk of cardiovascular mortality.

Since it came out, more than 80,000 diabetics who have been taking Avandia have suffered from a stroke, heart attack, or other serious cardiovascular complication.

Finally, after ten years of catastrophic use, the FDA finally restricted access to this drug.

Prescription Drugs and their Side Effects

Medication	Use For	Side Effects
Sulfonylureas *Includes Chlorpropamide Glimepiride Glipizide Glyburide Tolazamide Tolbutamide* *Brand names* • *Diabinese* • *Amaryl* • *Glucotrol* • *Glucotrol XL* • *DiaBeta* • *Glynase* • *PresTab* • *Micronase*	Lowering blood sugar levels by increasing pancreatic insulin production	• Extreme drops in blood sugar level • Stomach upset • Nausea • Increased appetite • Skin rash • Weight gain • Heightened susceptibility to sunburn • Hypoglycemia in the absence of food
Biguanides *Generic Name Metformin* *Brand names* • *Glucophage* • *Glucophage XR* • *Glumetza* • *Fortamet* • *Riomet*	Decreasing the need for insulin. Note: they do not increase insulin production	• Nausea • Abdominal gas • Diarrhea • Loss of appetite • Extreme tiredness • Dizziness • Menstruation may restart in post-menopausal women • Metallic taste • Low vitamin B12 levels Note: Never take with alcohol

Alpha-glucosidase inhibitors *Generic Name* Acarbose Miglitol *Brand names* • Precose • Glyset	Slowing down the rate of digestion of complex carbohydrates Note: they do not increase insulin production	• Gas • Bloating • Diarrhea • Stomach pain Note: you must take this medication with the first bit of food
Thiazolidinediones *Generic Names* Pioglitazone Rosiglitazone *Brand names* • Actos • Avandia	• Decreasing cell resistance to insulin • Decreasing glucose production by the liver	• Swelling in ankles, feet, and legs • Weight gain • Fluid retention which can lead to heart failure, anemia, head aches, nasal congestion • Higher risk of liver disease
Meglitinides *Generic Names* Nateglinide Repaglinide *Brand names* • Starlix Prandin	Controling post-eating blood-sugar spiking by increasing pancreatic insulin production	Hypoglycemia • Weight gain • Joint pain
DPP-4 Inhibitors *Generic Names* Linagliptin Saxagliptin *Brand names* • Tradjenta Onglyza	Prevents the DPP-4 enzyme from removing incretin from the body. Incretin is a signaler of insulin production.	• Nasal congestion • Upper respiratory infection • Painful urine • Bloody urine • Headache

IV. THE NASTY TRUTH ABOUT SUGAR

Are you addicted to sugar?

That fact that you're a human makes it highly likely. You see, the human body is hard-wired for sugar. Your taste buds are programmed to go crazy for it.

Every single one of the tens of thousands of taste bud receptors in your mouth have special sweetness receptors. Each of them are also connected to the brain's pleasure center. In effect, they receive a reward for satisfying the body's sugar fix.

But the craving isn't just in your taste buds. Recent research has discovered that sugar taste receptors are also located in the stomach, esophagus, and even the pancreas.

All of them are linked to your appetite.

When it comes to addiction, cocaine's got nothing on sugar. According to Dr. Pamela Peeke, author of The Hunger Fix, "Animal studies have shown that refined sugar is more addictive than cocaine, heroin, or morphine. An animal will choose an Oreo over morphine. Why? This cookie has the perfect combination of sugar and fat to hijack the brain's reward center."

For more than eighty years now, food manufacturers have been well aware of the human sugar addiction. They use this knowledge to increase their profit margins in countless ways.

- Sugar creates a consumer addiction to a manufacturer's product
- Sugar can make products fry up bigger and look puffier
- Sugar can prevent foods from going stale

As a result, sugar is in everything. What's so bad about that?

Glad you asked!

What Sugar is REALLY Doing to Your Body

Take a look at this list of immediate effects of putting too much sugar into your body:

- Chronic inflammation
- Premature aging
- Formation of free radicals
- Lower insulin production
- Pre-diabetes
- Increased risk of cancer
- Higher LDL cholesterol
- Hair loss and tooth decay
- ADHD
- Breakouts and skin irritations
- Obesity
- Allergies

- Hypertension
- Insomnia
- Depression
- Cardiovascular disease
- Creates acid overload
- Impairs liver function
- Mood swings and irritability
- Asthma
- Arthritis

Now, let's hone in on the six major effects that sugar is having on your health.

- Sugar can Make You Obese
- Sugar can Rot Your Teeth
- Sugar can Ruin Your Liver
- Sugar can Give You Diabetes
- Sugar Can Give You Cancer
- Sugar can Increase Your Chances of a Heart Attack

The problem with sugar is not the sugar itself. The problem is how much sugar you take in and how well equipped your body is to metabolize it.

Sugar is the gasoline of your body. Your body loves and needs sugar. Your physical body wouldn't exist if there wasn't sugar. In fact, sugar is so important to your body that your liver can make it. It does this through a process called gluconeogenesis.

So, the problem isn't sugar alone. The problem is when you consume too much sugar.

If you look at a chart for the amount of sugar we were eating in the 1800s and the amount of sugar we're eating now, you will be blown away. Our sugar consumption has skyrocketed.

One of the reasons for the huge uptake of sugar is that the foods we eat nowadays are grown in soil that is deficient in minerals. As a result, the food doesn't taste as good and the food industry pumps it with sugar to make it more palatable.

As a result, we are culturally consuming way too much sugar. Imagine that all the cells in your body are like tiny cars. They all need gasoline. To provide that fuel, sugar has to get inside the tank of all the cells in your body. It does that through the use of insulin.

When you eat something with sugar in it, there is sugar in your bloodstream. When there's sugar in the blood, the pancreas secretes insulin. Now there is both insulin and sugar in the blood. The insulin travels through the bloodstream and binds to insulin receptors on the outsides of each cell. This then sends a signal to the inside of the cell to open up a sugar door to allow the fuel that is the sugar into the cell.

However, in order for the signal to get from the insulin receptors on the outside of the cell to the inside where the door is opened to let the sugar in, certain key minerals and other nutrients need to be present within the cell. It they are not there, the door will remain permanently closed.

What happens to all the sugar? It piles up in the blood.

As a response to this, the body makes more insulin.

This is called Insulin Resistance Syndrome. It is also known as Syndrome X and Metabolic Syndrome.When insulin piles up in the bloodstream in huge amounts, by sheer volumetric pressure, it punches holes in the cell wall and the cell dies!

This is why people with diabetes sometimes get gangrene and lose their toes, fingers, and limbs.So, did you pick up what causes the failure of the mechanism that allows the sugar to enter the cell?

Lack of key minerals

The first of those key minerals is Chromium. In 1957, an M.D. by the name of Walter Mertz proved with scientific studies on mice just how crucial chromium is. When mice were deprived of chromium, they developed type 2 diabetes. When chromium was reintroduced, the diabetes went away. We'll discover more about the amazing diabetes-healing effects of chromium soon.

Becoming Sugar Aware

In order to gain mastery over sugar, you need to learn to observe how your body reacts to this sweet poison. Becoming sugar aware involves:

- Reading the labels: Become aware of the various names for sugar. Keep aware of the fact that the nearer an item is to the top of the list, the more of it there is in the product.
- Knowing what everyday foods you eat that are sugar loaded.
- Observing how your body reacts to sugar, especially fructose and high fructose corn syrup.
- Monitoring how you feel upon waking– do you feel like springing out of bed or like rolling over and going back to sleep?
- Monitoring your sense of taste and smell.
- Checking the color of your urine – the lighter the better.
- Getting a journal and recording your observations regarding sugar and how your body reacts to it.
- Going through your pantry and separating all the foods that contain an unhealthy level of sugar. Mark these items with

colored tape.
- Making a list of all the artificial sweeteners that you use. Mark these with another colored tape. If it contains both sugar and artificial sweeteners put both pieces of tape on it.
- Recruiting the other members of your family to support you in your quest to gain mastery over sugar.

Should You Take Artificial Sweeteners?

With the myriad problems associated with sugar, taking an artificial sweetener to get your daily fix may seem like a good idea. What you may not realize is that many of those sugar substitutes can actually be hazardous to your health. So, why are artificial sweeteners so bad for us?

The key is in the very name. Anything labelled artificial is usually created by a chemist in a laboratory. The resulting product cannot be easily digested by the body. In fact, study after study links these chemicals to imbalances created inside the body. This research has linked artificial sweeteners to:

- Depression
- Joint aches
- Alzheimer's disease
- Parkinson's disease
- Cancer
- Death

Furthermore, there is no concrete evidence to show that these sugar substitutes even help people to lose weight. On the contrary, studies show that chemical sweeteners can actually stimulate the appetite and lead to obesity.

Let's take a closer look at the common artificial sweeteners you're likely to run across:

Sucralose

Sucralose is made from real sugar that is chemically modified to be calorie free. They do this by adding chlorine. But that's not all. Other chemicals used in the manufacture of sucralose are acetone (a key ingredient of nail-polish remover), benzene (an ingredient used in oil and gasoline), methanol (used in windshield washer fluid) and formaldehyde (used to preserve dead bodies). Some of the chemicals used to make sucralose are listed on the US Environmental Protection Agency's list of most deadly poisons.

Aspartame

Aspartame is sometimes listed on food labels as phenylalanine. It has been the subject of a lot of heated controversy, both because of both safety issues and questionable circumstances surrounding its FDA approval. Aspartame is the cause of more complaints to the FDA than any other food. Aspartame use can lead to:

- Memory loss
- Headaches
- Dizziness
- Seizures
- Nausea
- Weight Gain

- Depression
- Insomnia
- Fatigue

This is just a partial list. Aspartame has ninety-two official side effects that have been reported to the FDA. One of them is Parkinson's Disease. In fact, many people believe that it was his constant exposure to Aspartame as a result of his endorsement of Diet Pepsi that led to Michael J. Fox's developing Parkinson's Disease at the unprecedented age of twenty-nine years. Still, Aspartame is used in over six thousand products worldwide. These include:

- Sodas
- Cereals
- Chewing Gum
- Desserts
- Breath mints
- Teas
- Coffees
- Yogurt

Saccharine

Throughout the 1960s and 70s studies showed that saccharine was linked to cancer in animals. In 1977, the FDA proposed a ban on this sugar substitute, but ended up issuing a warning label on the packet. Saccharine is a coal-tar derivative and has absolutely no food value. It is created by chemists in a laboratory.

One of the chemicals used to create saccharin is ammonia, which is also used for cleaning toilets. Other chemicals used to make saccharine are sulphur dioxide and chlorine. Common side effects are headaches, diarrhea, and hives.

Saccharine is often used to sweeten drinks. This causes even more problems for your body. When you gulp down your saccharine-sweetened soda, the pancreas responds by upping insulin production. In effect, your body is expecting food and getting prepared to digest it. But, unless you eat something with your soda, no food will accompany the liquid that has just gone down your throat. This will lead to a craving for high-carb food in order to allow the insulin to do its job. That's why saccharine has been linked to weight gain and obesity.

Acesulfame K

This sweetener is two hundred times sweeter than sucrose. It is made by chlorinating sugar. It has a negative impact on the thyroid. When your thyroid isn't working well, your metabolism is affected and you are not burning as many calories. One in five Americans are on thyroid medication, many of them as a result of their addiction to diet sodas that contain Acesulfame K. In 1988 Acesulfame K was listed as a potential substance that causes cancer by the Center for Science in the Public Interest after a number of studies showed a direct relation to the growth of tumors and leukemia in animals.

Agave

Agave contains calories, unlike the sweetenersmentioned above. Agave nectar is a natural sweetener produced from the agave plant.

The juice is extracted from the plant's core, filtered, heated, treated with enzymes, and then concentrated until it becomes a syrupy liquid.

The main problem with agave nectar is that it contains high levels of fructose. Studies have shown that high amounts of fructose in the body can promote triglyceride levels. High triglycerides are a known risk factor for heart disease. Eating fructose can also cause bloating, gas, and stomach discomfort. In addition, fructose is bad news for your liver.

High Fructose Corn Syrup (HFCS)

High fructose corn syrup is the most abundant sugar. The average American consumes about seventy pounds of it each year. In high fructose corn syrup, fructose and glucose are not chemically attached. The fructose is immediately delivered to your liver. It turns on a fat-production mechanism that can lead to fatty liver. It can also lead to:

- Heart disease
- Cancer
- Dementia
- Diabetes

There are also chemical contaminants in high fructose corn syrup. These include chlor-alkali, which contains mercury. With the average person consuming some twenty teaspoons a day of high fructose corn syrup, this can lead to a deadly buildup of mercury in the system.

High fructose corn syrup is a signal that the food which contains it is low quality. It will be processed and full of toxins that can destroy your health. You need to go into your kitchen and identify the foods that contain HFCS. Collect them all up in your arms and drop them into the garbage bin.

MSG

Monosodium glutamate is a flavor enhancer that is responsible for cranking up the sensation of savory flavors on our tongue. This flavor enhancement comes from an amino acid called L-Glutamate.

MSG is hidden in thousands of processed foods.

MSG has been associated with increased fat storage around the abdomen, increased risk of heart disease, osteoporosis, and diabetes. Look for products that contain MSG and avoid them at all costs.

White Bread

That loaf of bread that looks so appetizing is, in fact, a gooey, indigestible, and incomplete protein, a few multivitamins, and a whole lot of sugar. White bread, in particular, is problematic to the body. It's empty calories made with bleached flour and has all the nutrients stripped out of it. That's why most health conscious people pass by the white bread for a more wholesome alternative. In fact, many people are avoiding grains altogether and choosing paleo bread alternatives made mostly from nuts and eggs. Paleo breads are naturally high in protein and fiber and low in calories.

White Rice

We associate white rice with healthy food. We think of it as a great source of complex carbs. Of course, it's a staple of Asian diet. Yet, recent research indicates that white rice may be linked to type 2 diabetes.

Harvard researchers found that people who eat white rice are one and a half times more likely to develop type 2 diabetes than those who ate minimal amounts. In one study, the risk of diabetes increased 10 percent for every extra bowl of white rice consumed. This study was published in the British Medial Journal on March 15, 2012 (2).

The problem with white rice is that it is high on the glycemic index and will spike your blood sugar levels.

By now, there's no doubt that sugar, both real and artificial, is toxic to your body. But, unless you can find a replacement in order to satisfy your sweet tooth, you are destined to failure. Fortunately, there are alternatives available that are safe, healthy and, above all, tasty. These are your new friends. So, let's get you acquainted:

Stevia

Stevia is an herb that originates in South America. It has been used as a sweetener for hundreds of years. Stevia is three hundred times sweeter than sugar and has a delicious and refreshing taste.

Because the body does not break down the glycosides contained in stevia, it has no calories. In addition, stevia enhances insulin secretion without adversely affecting blood glucose levels. It also produces anti- hyperglycemic properties.

Stevia can be purchased as whole or broken leaves. It is also available in powder form and as a liquid extract. Dried stevia keeps its flavor for months. Use one teaspoon in place of one cup of sugar. It is available under such brand names such as Truvia, Nu Naturals and Sweetleaf. You can buy pure stevia as a dietary supplement. Many brands of stevia have added flavorings, indicating that they have been highly processed. Make sure that you check the label!

Because stevia is so potent, you don't have to use very much of it. Purchase it in small amounts until you find a brand that you enjoy. Often the taste is disagreeable because people use too much of it. If you need more sweetness add one drop at a time and then taste it.

Stevia has few side effects. Studies investigating any potential links between liver disorders and cancer have concluded that, unless used excessively, stevia is safe. However, it may lower your blood sugar. That's why it's important that your use of stevia goes hand in hand with a clean, healthy diet in which sugar has been eliminated. You should be consuming plenty of natural carbs, proteins, and fats. And you should be eating every four waking hours.

Honey

Honey is nature's healthy alternative to sugar. Not only is it safe and delicious but it contains some major health benefits. It is an antibacterial, antiviral superfood. It can also help you to fight allergies, improve your immune system, fight cancer, and even lower cholesterol. Studies have also shown that honey helps to fight diabetes. It turns out that honey contains a perfect one-to-one ratio of glucose to fructose, facilitating glucose intake into the liver and overcoming excess blood sugar.

You need to be consuming honey every day in order to conquer your diabetes.

Fruit

Natural, whole fruits contain all of the sweetness you need, without any of the toxic chemicals that will poison your body. Oranges contain a delectable juiciness, ripe strawberries create a sweet symphony in your mouth, and blended frozen bananas serve up all the richness of ice- cream – without the guilt. Dried fruit offers sweetness plus fiber.

It's all a matter of mindset. Once you step away from the mindset of having to add artificial flavorings to your foods, a whole new world of healthy food appreciation will open to you. And you'll finally be able to gain mastery over your taste buds.

V. THE REAL WAY TO DROP THE EXCESS WEIGHT

Fear of saturated fats and cholesterol is everywhere. We are constantly bombarded with advertising convincing us to lower our cholesterol levels by not eating saturated fat. We're also being given drugs, called statins, that are designed to lower cholesterol and, therefore, reduce the risk of having a heart attack.

The problem is that these approaches to improving our cardiovascular health are misguided. In this section, we will investigate the two recommendations that the drug companies base their approach to weight and cholesterol control upon:

(1) Limiting cholesterol and saturated fat consumption

(2) Keeping serum cholesterol levels as low as possible

We'll discover that the conventional view of fat and cholesterol is inaccurate – and find out what you really have to do to reduce yourweight and benefit your cardiovascular health.

Some Diet History

The first recorded modern account of an overweight person trying to shed pounds was William Banting (1797 – 1878). Banting's doctor recommended a low- carbohydrate diet that eliminated such things as potatoes, bread, and sugar. He was able to eat as much meat and animal products as he desired.

This approach was very successful, with Banting losing forty-six pounds, and living into his 80s. He went on to write a book in which he detailed what he ate to achieve his weight loss. Banting's take-home message was that reducing carbs was the key to weight loss.

A few years later, doctors in the US began turning their attention to the problem of weight gain. In the late nineteenth century, Dr. Emmet Densmore wrote a book arguing against consumption of grains and starchy foods. Just like Banting, Densmore stated that obesity is caused by foods high in carbohydrates.

During the 1950s, Alfred Pennington became a leader in the field of obesity study. In one of his manypapers, Pennington recommended that people should eat a half pound or more of fresh meat with the fat every day.

Pennington further stated that most of the meat people buy is not fatty enough, so they should buy extra beef fat. Not only that, but he urged readers to eat as much of this food as they wanted.

In harmony with his predecessors, Pennington advised avoiding bread, flour, and sugar. Then came Dr. Robert Atkins in 1972, with his book Diet Revolution. Formany people, Atkin's ideas seemed revolutionary. But as we've seen, the weight-loss method of avoiding carbohydrates instead of fat is nothing new. In fact, for more than a century, research has shown it's the carbohydrates that make you fat – and that eating fat is actually healthy.

Is It Healthy to Eat Low Carbs and High Fat?

One hundred fifty years of research has established that, contrary to generally accepted wisdom, it is healthy to eat a high-fat diet.

A 2006 study by Dashi et al showed that not only was a high fat, low-carb diet effective at reducing body fat, it also reduced all of the significant biomarkers. HDL (good cholesterol) went up, fats in the blood went down, and blood glucose drops dramatically.

In 2015, the Journal Nutrition cited the work of more than two hundred scholars who emphasized that carb restriction is the ideal approach to treating type 2 diabetes, obesity, and cardiovascular disease.

So, 150 years of research confirms that carbohydrates are the demon on your plate. Why, then are so many of us still so fat and cholesterol averse?

The reason is that, despite the overwhelming evidence to the contrary, the American Heart Association, dietitians, and nutritionists are demonizing fat. To lose weight, they say, we need to be eating fat free.

Why the Low-Fat Mania?

These recommendations are completely out of touch with the science. How can this be?

The low-fat food mania began in 1955 when President Eisenhower had a heart attack. This incident highlighted the growing incidences of Americans having heart attacks.

Everyone ignored the fact that Americans, including their President, had become chain smokers. Instead, it was claimed that what was killing Eisenhower was the sausage he was eating with breakfast. Fat in the diet was pinpointed as the cause of weight gain and heart attacks.

The Rise of Ancel Keys

In 1953, Ancel Keys, the man behind the "fat is bad" myth, published a newsletter in which he proposed a relationship between fat in the diet and people dying of heart attacks.

However, Keys manipulated his data to make it appear that fat consumption was related to obesity. He had twenty-two countries to draw data from, but hand picked six of them to back up his claims, ignoring the other sixteen. When you look at all of the data, you realize that there is, in fact, no relationship between fat in the diet and heart disease.

Despite this, Ancel Keys became the leader of nutrition and cardiovascular research in America. It was he who popularized the notion that Americans eat too much fat. Keys became such a dominant figure in the American Heart Association that its current recommendations still follow Key's original faulty ideas.

Keys is the father of the Mediterranean Diet, advocating that we eat just 15 percent of our overall calories from fat and only 4 percent from saturated fat. However, studies in the 2000s actually show that more fat in the diet is correlated with fewer incidences of heart disease – the direct opposite to what Keys had claimed.

The French Paradox

In a study published in the 2012 British Journal of Nutrition, a comparison was made between countries related to obesity and heart attack. The country which had the lowest incidence of heart attack was the very country that ate the most saturated fat– France. French people eat 40 percent fat, of which 15 percent is saturated fat (4).

Because the results from France ran counter to the hypothesis created by Keys, it was labelled a paradox.

The well-known Food Pyramid was developed by the US Dept. of Agriculture. It advocated a high-carb, low-fat diet. This is what guided what people ate in the 1970s and 1980s. The result was that people gained weight.

Americans got bigger as a result of the demonization of fat. Fortunately, good science ultimately prevails. As a result, in the last five years, the message became clearer that carbs are the problem, not fat. Studies are now coming out, one after the other, showing that the guidance based on Keys' theory is wrong.

What About the Keto Diet?

If you thought the world had been turned upside down when Donald Trump was elected POTUS, spare a thought for the "fat is bad" crusaders of the last thirty years. Their mantra has been turned on its head as millions of people jump onto the ketogenic bandwagon and pile their plates with fried bacon, sausages, and butter in an attempt to consume as much fat as they can.

Is there any method in this madness or is it just the latest in a long line of off-the-wall fat-loss gimmicks?

How We Got Here

The Ketogenic diet is nothing new. Its concept of a high fat, moderate protein, and very low carb diet has been around for more than 150 years. In fact, until the 1950s, it was the go-to fat-loss method advocated by the mainstream medical community.

It wasn't until 1955, in the wake of President Eisenhower's heart attack, that fat began to be demonized. Since then, the official line has been to get out the fat and pump up the carbs. All we need to do is look around us to see what the results have been.

It's no exaggeration to say that the low-fat, high-carb way of eating has been a disaster. As a direct result of it, we are heavier, more sedentary, and more likely to die from fatal illness.

A Return to Keto

The Ketogenic diet is designed to switch your primary energy system from a carbohydrate to a fat source. By switching over from a carb-based glucose to a fat-based ketone fuel system, you will be actually burning stored body fat as your main way to provide your body with the energy that it needs to function.

When the acids in fats are broken down during the digestive process, they become ketones. This can either be used as energy or stored as reserve energy in the form of body fat.

On a conventional high-carb diet, the energy contained in the carbs becomes glucose in the body. This is what the body first turns to in order to get the energy that it needs to function. However, when carb intake is restricted, the body will turn to its secondary energy supply –

ketones.

Achieving the state of ketosis – when the body is relying on ketones as its energy source – is the goal of the ketogenic diet.

Keto Beats Cravings

A major side effect of eating carbs is that it releases the storage hormone insulin. As well as storing 10 percent of your ingested carbs as fat for a pending time of famine, insulin also causes sharp fluctuations in your blood-sugar levels. This leads to cravings – the Achilles heel of anyone who's tried to lose weight!

However, when you switch to a high-fat diet, you will no longer be releasing insulin every time you eat. As a result, you won't be piling on that 10 percent of fat storage

– and you won't get the sugar cravings that come with carbs.

In addition, a high-fat diet is extremely filling. A meal of sausages, fried eggs, and tomatoes will fill you up for at least four hours. That is because it is fat, not carbs or protein, that triggers feelings of satiation.

So, Does It Work?

The keto revival has been underway for around twenty years. There are literally millions of people the world over who can relate their experiences of just how successful it is at losing weight. In addition, there are scores of peer-reviewed scientific studies that show just how effective a ketogenic diet is at lowering body fat levels.

In fact, it is safe to say that following a ketogenic eating pattern is the fastest, most effective and safest way to lose body fat that exists.

Yet the benefits of keto go well beyond its ability to strip body fat. The Keto diet can also . . .

- Control type 2 diabetes
- Fight cancer
- Target visceral body fat
- Lower triglyceride levels
- Give you more energy

The keto diet is for real. In fact, it's not really a diet at all – keto is an eating pattern that should form the foundation of your nutritional approach for the rest of your life.

Keto and Diabetes

Type 2 diabetes is a dietary disease caused by too much sugar. The key to controlling it is to cut out all of the sugar and refined carbohydrates. The ketogenic diet does exactly that by restricting carbs to less than 20 grams per day. One form of the keto diet is espoused by the American Diabetes Association.

There are three macronutrients in the typical human diet: carbohydrates, fats, and proteins. Of these three, carbs are the only macronutrients that dramatically spike blood glucose levels. Protein raises it a little and fat doesn't raise it at all. It only makes sense, then, to consume a very low- carbohydrate, adequate-protein, and high- fat diet. That is what keto does.

Yet, the general medical community recommendations when advising type

2 diabetics is to consume 40-65 grams of carbohydrates per meal, plus extras through snacks.

That's a lot of carbs.

All of those carbs are going to shoot blood sugar levels through the roof. In otherwords, doctors are recommending that people eat exactly what is causing their problems.

If that sounds crazy, that's because it is!

At its root, diabetes is a state of carbohydrate toxicity. We can't get the blood sugar into the cells. That causes a problem in the short term but the long term consequences are even greater.

Insulin resistance is basically a state of carbohydrate intolerance. So, why would we want to continue to recommend to people to eat carbs?

The American Diabetes Association guidelines specifically state that there is insufficient evidence to recommend a specific carb limit. But those guidelines go right on to say that carbohydrate intake is the single biggest factor in blood sugar levels.

The American Diabetes Association guidelines go on to state that if you're taking certain diabetic medications then you need to take in more carbs, otherwise your blood sugar levels could get too low.

In other words, people eat too many carbs, so they have to take medicine. Then they have to eat more carbs to avoid the side effects of those medicines. This creates a crazy, vicious cycle which will have you eating more and more carbs, while getting heavier and going more and more into a diabetic state.

The truth is that we DO NOT need carbohydrates at all.

Our essential daily requirement for carbs is ZERO.

We have essential amino acids (proteins), essential fatty acids, but no essential carbs.

A nutrient is essential if we have to have it to function and we can't make it from something else. Yet, the body makes plenty of glucose all the time through gluconeogenesis.

So, if we don't need much in the way of carbs, and the consumption of them is making us sick, why are our so called "experts" recommending that we take in more than half of our daily energy requirements in the form of carbohydrates?

When you decrease your carbs, your glucose goes down. As a result, you won't need as much insulin. The insulin levels will then drop – fast.

A recent study that looked at United States National Health and Nutrition Examination Survey data showed that the single biggest risk factor for coronary artery disease is insulin resistance. It is responsible for a whopping 42 percent of heart attacks (5).

Low-carb intervention works so fast that hundreds of people can be pulled off of insulin in days.

The Keto diet, of course, is something that the Vedda people of Sri Lanka have never come across. Yet, it is amazing how similar the native Vedda diet is to the Keto diet. Of course, the Vedda do not eat processed carbohydrate foods. Their diet is high in protein and fat. They don't trim the fat off their meats and they get a lot of healthy fats through foods like coconut.

The Vedda actually eat more protein than most people who are on a keto diet, so the ideal Vedda-based way of eating is more closely aligned to a modern paleo diet than a keto diet. Paleo emphasizes the nutrient- dense food that the human body thrives on, while eliminating the highly processed refined foods that have become the mainstay of the modern Western diet.

The Paleo Diet is built around the following foods:

- Meat
- Fish
- Fruits
- Vegetables
- Nuts and Seeds
- Starchy Plants

And those are the very food types that the Vedda have been consuming for the last three thousand years!

To the above list we can add the following recommendations:

- If it says lite, low fat or fat free, leave it in the grocery store. You can be sure that if they took the fat out, they put carbs and chemicals in.
- Eat FOOD – real food does not come in a box and no one needs to tell you that real food is natural – you should know that when you look at it.
- Don't eat anything you don't like.
- Eat when you're hungry and don't eat when you're not.
- NO GPS – grains, potatoes, or sugars
- Use non-grain based flours – especially coconut flour, but also use almond, hazelnut, and flax

By analyzing different low-carb diet options, we have built a highly effective diabetes- defeating long-term diet plan. It provides us with a springboard into the Vedda diet.

VI. WISDOM OF THE VEDDA

In order to fully appreciate just how we can benefit from the 3000-year-old knowledge of the Vedda people, we need to take a closer look at this fascinating culture. By doing so, we'll be able to isolate the lifestyle and dietary factors that have led them to be the only population in the world that has never had a recorded case of diabetes.

The Vedda are native inhabitants of Sri Lanka, which is located off the southern tip of India. The word Vedda means hunter, a fitting representation of these jungle- dwelling people. They are widely referred to as forest dwellers and it is generally accepted that they are descended from Neolithic ancestors. The origins of the Vedda have been recorded in a sacred manuscript which is known as The Mahavamsa, roughly translated as "The Great Chronicle."

According to the Mahavamsa, Sri Lanka's first king married a beautiful but devilish woman by the name of Kuveni. The royal couple had two children. Before long, though, the king abandoned his queen and children and married a lovely Indian princess of noble birth.

The abandoned Kuveni was put to death by her own relatives. But, the two boys escaped to the remote jungle mountains. Their descendants became the Vedda people. Their dead mother, Kuveni, is worshipped even today as the Maha Loku Kiriammaleththo (Great Mother).

Three thousand years later, the Vedda have been untouched by time. They still cling to their ancient tribal ways, refusing to be contaminated by the encroachment of modern society. This is even more remarkable given the vehement attempts of every Sri Lankan ruling class to colonize them. Of course, some – mainly young men – have drifted off to metropolitan areas to be consumed by the system, but the vast majority have remained true to their heritage.

Today the Vedda people can be demographically classed into three groups:

- the Bintenne Veddas
- the Anuradhapura Veddas
- the Coast Veddas

The three groups are geographically isolated from one another across the jungle regions of Sri Lanka, having very little contact. There are believed to be about 6,600 Vedda in Sri Lanka, against a total Sri Lankan population of 20.48 million.

Theirs is a matriarchal society with lineage being traced only through the female line of descent. There is no concept of masculinity among the Vedda, with women having an equal status in all things.

Hunting is the main preoccupation of Vedda men. They consider the tracking and killing of all creatures to be a sacred endeavor. They hunt with the bow and arrow on land and use the harpoon on the water. They also use toxic plants to kill their prey.

The Vedda people will only kill a creature if they need to eat it.

The Vedda speak their own language, which is a unique and pure grammatical core. The Vedda are a spiritual people and follow a system of worship that can be categorized as a blend of Animism and Totemism. They believe that certain plants and animals possess special powers. They also worship ancestors who have died.

The Vedda Diet

The Vedda are well known for following a diet that is very rich in meat. Main meats that are eaten are venison, rabbit, turtle, tortoise, monitor lizard, wild boar, and the brown monkey. They also eat a lot of fish.

The Vedda enjoy a special delicacy known as gona perume. This is a type of sausage, which contains alternate layers of fat and meat. Another favorite dish is goya-tel- perume, which is the tailof the monitorlizard, stuffed with fat and roasted on embers. Dried meat preserve soaked in honey is yet another delicacy that the Vedda indulge in.

Vedda cultivate yams, coconut, maize, melons and gourds.

Amongst every Vedda tribe can be find at least one medicine man who has a working knowledge of ancient Ayurvedic medicine. Healing is done with the aid of herbal concoctions. However, some conditions are thought to be the result of demonic possession, with the only remedy being exorcism.

Lakmal's Account

Do you remember Lakmal?

He was the old man that I met in a hospital waiting room that fateful day when I was accompanying Rachel on a routine check up. Lakmal was 91 years old and was with his wife, who needed a hip replacement.

Despite their years, they both appeared to be in their sixties. They had a healthy glow about them that you very rarely see – and NEVER see in people in their nineties.

Lakmal was the man who turned to me and said, "I come from a place where diabetes doesn't even exist, and it's because of the food we eat."

Since that day, I've enjoyed many phone conversations with Lakmal. I soon realized the value of what he was telling me and, so that I didn't forget any of it, I began taping our conversations (with his permission of course). What follows is the actual transcript of one of our calls.

I can remember in childhood our village was surrounded by jungle. Where the sun went up, the sunshine did not reach us as the jungle was so thick. We had enough animals to hunt and we had enough space to grow our crops.

Everybody lived very peacefully. I was the leader of our tribe, just as my father had been. The real story of the Vedda is different to the one in the history books. They say that the Vedda came from India three thousand years ago. But the real story is that we have been here for ten thousand years. Only seven hundred people came here from India to escape their troubles.

The Vedda moved into the forest. All the land belongs to them. When we lived in the jungle we never went to school. We were educated by the jungle. People were free to do what they wanted and be their own person. There was no pressure to be someone else. Our hunters would go out and stalk their prey, bringing back their kill slung over their shoulder.

When I was a child, I believed my home to be a paradise. There was no sickness, no fevers, nobody ever died in childbirth. There were no overweight people. And there was never anything called diabetes.

It was only when I moved to America that I learned about these sicknesses. I couldn't believe all the overweight people that I saw. I soon made the connection with the food they were eating. Actually, I called it "not food" because it was not grown from the earth or killed. The food that people eat in America is grown in a laboratory. It is no wonder that diabetes is such a big problem.

Imagine the difference between living under the trees and going back to the cities. Under a tree you will feel something different. Nature provides everything you need. In town you may feel hungry, but food is not free. You have to go to a fast food place and pay for it – and it is not even real food.

In the jungle, everything is free. Rain, oxygen, food, shelter; everything you would ever need.

That was just one of many taped accounts from Lakmal. Yet, can't you just hear his simple wisdom shining through? Lakmal was well aware of the hypocrisy of the modern western world. We look at jungle dwellers such as the Vedda people and immediately tell ourselves that we've got to save them. We have to introduce them to the 21st century, to bring them to the best way of life.

Of course, the reality is that they already have the best way of life. And they are the ones who can help us to find the better way.

After all, they are not in the midst of an obesity epidemic. They are not the ones whose children are dying from diabetes . . .

We are!

So, lets learn from these amazing people and take charge of our own bodies and our own lives.

Summary

The Vedda have lived for thousands of years in the jungles of Sri Lanka, thriving on a simple way of life that revolves around hunting, fishing, and growing crops. Their diet consists of a lot of protein in the form of such meats as:

- venison
- rabbit
- turtle
- tortoise
- monitor lizard
- wild boar
- brown monkey

The Vedda also eat a lot of slow-release carb vegetables and fruits that are full of vitamins and fiber. Their main sources are:

- yams
- maize
- melons
- gourds
- coconut

It's no surprise that the diet of the Vedda is virtually identical to what Western medical experts are now advocating for a diabetes- free lifestyle. When it comes to type 2 diabetes, we need to balance our blood sugar. Diet-wise there are certain foods that will help to do that. It is recommended that meals be high in the following:

- Protein
- Fiber
- Healthy Fat

Those three things will go a long way in helping to balance out your blood sugar levels. The things that will throw it all off track are sugar and carbs. You do need carbohydrates, but only in small amounts. You will also want to ingest foods that are very high in the mineral chromium. One food that contains a whole lot of chromium, along with plenty of fiber, is broccoli.

Foods that are rich in magnesium have also been shown to be hugely beneficial. Magnesium has also been shown to help control blood-sugar levels. That is why grass-fed beef, and many types of nuts, seeds, and vegetables are great for fighting diabetes.

Western science has also come to appreciate the vital need for fiber when combating diabetes. And, of course there is now a growing appreciation for the amazing diabetic healing properties of coconut oil. Coconut oil is great for burning fat and controlling blood-sugar levels.

The experts are also advocating lots of protein. Wild-caught salmon seems to be the protein of the moment, but grass-fed beef, organic chicken, and turkey are also good choices.

So far, have you noticed the similarities between what the Vedda people have been consuming for many centuries and what the modern day Western experts are now advocating?

It's pretty hard to miss, right?

After all, they're virtually indistinguishable.

The Vedda have been eating high protein, lots of fiber, and generous servings of healthy fats as a natural part of their existence for thousands of years. And, of course, those essential minerals such as chromium and magnesium came directly out of the soil.

Nobody told them they have to eat that way. It was what their environment produced and so it was what they ate.

Yet, it proved to be the perfect way to eat.

As a result, there has NEVER been a case of diabetes among these people.

Another notable lesson that we can learn from the Vedda is that they lead peaceable, stress-free lives. They follow the maxim embodied by the Bobby McFerrin song "Don't Worry, Be Happy." As a result, their blood pressure is not elevated, their sleep is not interrupted and they are not drawn to eating sugar-laden carb foods (if they could even find them!).

The lesson?

Learn to destress – it will allow you to find flow in your life. You'll be able to live more in the moment rather than also focusing on the destination.

And you'll be far happier.

VII. THE SECRET INGREDIENTS OF THE VEDDA THAT ELIMINATE DIABETES

Coconut

Coconuts are a truly amazing gift from nature that native peoples have been using as a staple to keep them healthy and vigorous for centuries. The Vedda people absolutely love coconuts and include the milk or pulp in virtually everything they eat.

The Western world is finally starting to embrace the power of the coconut for general wellbeing and enhanced longevity. But, most people still haven't fully realized that coconut is a wonder compound when it comes to combatting diabetes.

The coconut is so abundant in its healing properties, it is referred to as the tree of life. Prior to WWII, people living in island nations ate a diet that consisted mainly of rice, root crops, vegetables, and an abundance of this ultra-healing super food, the coconut.

The coconut is a functional food, being rich in vitamins, mineral and fiber – the essential nutritional building blocks for perfect health.

For generations, the Vedda people of the jungles of Sri Lanka considered the coconut the "cure for all illnesses." They have, and still do, consume the meat, milk and oil of the coconut on a daily basis.

Even though this diet is high in saturated fat, Western conditions such as diabetes, cancer, and heart disease are unheard of there. Instead, the Vedda people are rewarded with a lovely complexion, soft, wrinkle-free skin, and virtually no skin cancer – even with daily exposure to the sun. They enjoy natural good health and the vast majority of them are fully active well into their nineties.

Coconut oil has been shown to provide protection from viruses, bacteria, infections, thyroid cancer, and brain and heart problems. As a bonus it beautifies the skin – and even burns fat!

Coconut fiber has been found to have an almost magical ability to bring down blood sugar levels. When you consume carbohydrates, they are converted into glucose or blood sugar. Diabetics and pre-diabeticsare encouraged to consume foods that have a low glycemic index. The higher the glycemic index, the greater impact the food has on increasing blood sugar. (6)

The body knows that elevated blood sugar is a bad thing, and, in order to counterbalance it, it starts pumping insulin into the bloodstream to get things under control.

When you consume coconut oil, it slows down the absorption of sugars into the bloodstream. In this way it helps to balance blood sugar. It also helps the pancreas to secrete insulin and increase insulin sensitivity. Coconut oil is a powerful force to reverse insulin resistance.

Coconut oil even helps to improve the circulation of the blood in your body. Ironically, many people think that coconut oil will clog the arteries and slow down your circulation. In fact, it does just the opposite. (7)

One of the primary symptoms of diabetes is lack of circulation in the legs and feet. This was, in fact, one of the first things that my wife, Rachel, noticed – she'd lost the feeling in her legs and feet. Yet, within just a few days of going onto coconut oil, she'd got it all back.

As she so clearly demonstrated, coconut oil can improve circulation to the point that normal feeling returns. One man who I've recently introduced to the healing power of coconut oil told me that his legs had been numb for six years as a result of his diabetes. When this man received a cut in his lower leg, as a result of poor circulation, the cut refused to heal itself. It stayed the same for several months, showing absolutely no signs of healing.

I put this man on two to three tablespoons of coconut oil every day. Within ten days, the cut was completely healed and the circulation within his feet was restored. He had his normal feeling back – after six long years.

So, coconut oil has hugely beneficial aspects for diabetics. It is way better than eating corn oils or other types of oil. In fact, there is no herb or medicine that can reverse the effects of diabetes as effectively as coconut oil.

Coconut oil is excellent for keeping blood sugar under control. In fact, if you do happen to eat a meal that shoots your blood sugar up too high, simply take a couple of tablespoons of coconut oil. Within thirty minutes your blood sugar levels will have returned to normal.

Cinnamon

You may think of cinnamon as being a modern world herb that is used to add flavor to recipes. That's pretty much how I viewed it, too. So, I was somewhat surprised when Lakmal explained to me that the Vedda cultivate cinnamon and use it liberally for its heath giving properties.

Cinnamon comes from the inner layer of bark from several varieties of evergreen trees in Sri Lanka and South India. This beautiful spice smells and tastes great. It's magic for healing from diabetes because cinnamon reduces your blood sugar response to food. Over time it will actually improve your body's sensitivity to insulin. This means that your body doesn't have to produce as much insulin to get the sugar out of the blood.

Remember that the basic problem with diabetes is that your body doesn't respond to insulin anymore. That's why it is called insulin resistance – your body is resistant to insulin. As you already know, insulin is vital because it acts like a chaperone to take sugar out of your blood and into your body's cells. If sugar doesn't get into your cells, your blood sugar levels remain elevated, which is dangerous for your health.

Elevated blood sugar can damage the blood vessels around your eyes and lead to blindness. In a similar way, the nerves in your limbs are adversely affected, which can lead to loss of body parts.

Cinnamon will help your body to become sensitive to insulin once again.

Physicians have long been intrigued by the beneficial effects of cinnamon. In December 2003, an excellent study was published in Diabetes Care. In this study, the investigators divided a total of 60 type 2 diabetic patients into six groups. Groups 1, 2, and 3 were given cinnamon powder in a daily dose of 1 gram, 3 grams, and 6 grams respectively. Groups 4, 5, and 6 received placebo capsules. At the end of 40 days, there was a decrease of 18 - 29 percent in fasting blood glucose in cinnamon-treated patients, as compared with placebo groups. (8)

In addition, cinnamon also decreased serum triglycerides by 23 to 30 percent. Patients consuming 6 grams of cinnamon powder appeared to have achieved results earlier, but by 40 days, all doses had the same efficacy.

Neem

The Neem tree is an evergreen that is native to the Indian subcontinent, and is also found in the jungles of Sri Lanka. It is claimed that the oil, leaves, and bark of the Neem tree can treat forty different diseases. The Vedda people have been using it for thousands of years.

Among Neem's health promoting qualities are cancer fighting compounds and anti- oxidants that combat bladder infections and gum disease. For diabetics, Neem has been shown to reduce insulin requirements by up to 50 percent without altering blood- glucose levels. They do this by stimulating the beta-cells in the pancreas to produce insulin.

Neem also acts as a whole body detoxifier and helps to improve circulation. Look for Neem in the form of teabags, taking two cups daily.

Ginger

The Vedda people have been making use of the root of the ginger plant for centuries in order to relieve digestive issues and improve general health. They may not have been aware if it, but it has also been a huge factor in warding off diabetes.

In recent years, there has been a great interest in the medical community about the health benefits of ginger. Researchers are not entirely sure exactly how ginger works to improve diabetes. They do know that it contains such compounds as shogaols, paradols, and zingerone. These have all been shown to have anti-diabetic properties and strong antioxidant properties.

Recently, there have been a number of studies, animal as well as human, showing tremendous health benefits of ginger for diabetes, arthritis, cancer, and cardiovascular health.

For example, in an excellent study, researchers enrolled 88 type-2 diabetic patients. They divided them into two groups: ginger group and placebo group. The ginger group received ginger as 3 one-gram capsules daily for 8 weeks. The placebogroupreceived 3 one-gramdummy capsules daily for 8 weeks. At the end of 8 weeks, there was a significant decrease in fasting blood glucose, hemoglobin A1c, and insulin resistance in the group that received ginger. (9)

In another study, researchers enrolled 70 Type-2 diabetic patients and divided them into two groups. One group received a daily dose of 1600 mg ginger, while the other group received 1600 mg of placebo for 12 weeks. (10)

Compared with the placebo group, ginger significantly reduced fasting blood glucose, hemoglobin A1c, insulin resistance, triglyceride, total cholesterol, CRP (C-Reactive Protein), and PGE2 (Prostaglandin E2). CRP and PGE2 are markers for inflammation, which is extremely common in diabetic patients and indicates risk for cardiovascular events such as heart attack and stroke.

The Minerals that will Help Defeat Your Diabetes

Chromium

Because the Vedda people of Sri Lanka live in one of few remaining pristinely untouched areas of the world, most of the foods that they put into their bodies are filled with minerals derived from the soil.

That is in stark contrast with the rest of us. Our soils have been hugely depleted over the last century. They've been stripped of all of their mineral goodness as we've more heavily relied upon modern intensive agricultural methods. In a landmark 2004 study, conducted by the University of Texas, nutritional data were analyzed from 43 different vegetables and fruits from both 1950 and 1999. There was an overwhelming decline in the amounts of protein, calcium, phosphorus, chromium, iron, riboflavin and Vitamin C in the more recent group.

So, a major difference between the Vedda people and us is that they are still getting a full complement of minerals in their diets and we aren't. In fact, it has been estimated that 90 percent of the US population are chromium deficient. And it's not only soil deficiency which is responsible.

The high consumption of carbs, especially sugar drinks in the diet, will increase your chromium loss by 300 percent. So, every time you drink an 8-ounce glass of orange juice, apple juice, or soda, your body will expel a whole lot of chromium in your urine for the next twelve hours.

Chromium used to be called GTF, which stands for Glucose Tolerance Factor. This is a combination of chromium 3, d-nicotinic acid, and glutathione. GTF actually mimics insulin. So, it transports glucose from the outside of the cell to the inside of the cell.

Chromium deficiency is a major cause of the development of diabetes. Fasting plasma chromium levels are usually very low in pregnant women. It's believed that the impairment of chromium is what leads to the well-known cravings that most women experience during pregnancy.

Chromium deficiency is accelerated by vanadium deficiency.

Chromium's effect on blood-sugar levels was first discovered more than half a century ago. When researchers tested pre-diabetic rats with chromium, they found that it dramatically improved tolerance. It was at that time that chromium was labelled as Glucose Tolerance Factor (GTF). Since then, chromium has been widely studied for its effect on insulin.

One of the key effects of type 2 diabetes is insulin resistance. This means that the body doesn't respond properly to insulin. In more than a dozen studies, supplementation with glucose was found to improve glucose uptake in people with impaired glucose tolerance. When used in conjunction with biotin, it was shown to improve beta-cell function and glucose uptake and reduce glucose output from the liver.

In one study out of China, patients with type 2 diabetes were put into two groups. One group was given 200 mg of chromium per day. The other group was given 1000 mg daily. This resulted in statistically significant reductions in blood sugar levels. In the group that was taking 1000 mg per day, there was a 19 percent reduction in blood sugar levels. (11)

Chromium regulates insulin and prevents glucose levels from going either too high or too low. It also reduces fat storage to aid in weight loss. Chromium helps to maintain muscle mass and reduce sugar cravings. It has also been shown to convert sugar into energy in the body, lower fasting blood-sugar levels, lower insulin levels, and lower cholesterol.

The bottom line here is that you need to increase your dietary intake of chromium- rich foods. **Here are the best dietary sources:**

- Broccoli
- Oysters
- Salmon
- Turkey
- Liver
- Onions
- Eggs
- Seafood

In studies, chromium picolinate was shown to be the most effective form of supplemental chromium. Taking between 200 and 400 mcg per day is the recommended dosage for best results.

Several studies have shown beneficial effects of chromium supplementation in diabetic patients. In one such study, researchers investigated the effect of Chromium picolinate in Chinese individuals with type 2 diabetes. For four months, one group received Chromium picolinate 100 micrograms twice a day, the second group received Chromium picolinate 500 micrograms twice a day, and the third group received a placebo. (12)

Researchers noted significant improvements in glucose control as evidenced by fasting blood glucose, post-meal blood glucose and Hemoglobin A1c in the diabetics receiving 500 micrograms twice per day. There were fewer improvements in the group receiving 100 micrograms twice per day. In addition, there was improvement in insulin resistance and cholesterol level.

In another study, researchers evaluated twenty-five randomized, controlled trials and concluded that chromium supplementation, at a dose of more than 200 micrograms per day, has a favorable effect on glucose control in diabetic patients. In addition, Chromium picolinate appears to lower triglycerides and raise HDL cholesterol (the good cholesterol), by decreasing insulin resistance. Overall, chromium supplementation was found to be safe. (13)

Magnesium

Magnesium has been referred to as the twin of insulin. **So, what does it do?**

Magnesium is a basic building block of life. It is a very important factor for enzymes that are involved in carbohydrate metabolism. Magnesium and insulin are like twins who need each other. Without insulin, magnesium does not get transported from the blood to the cells. And without magnesium beta-cells will not secrete enough insulin, or the insulin it they do secrete will not be effective.

As a result of this co-dependent relationship, magnesium deficiency can lead to both the development of type 1 and type 2 diabetes.

Magnesium will decrease insulin transport and storage. It will also decrease insulin secretion. In addition, it will increase insulin resistance, and it will lead to what is called impaired glucose tolerance (IGT).

Magnesium deficiency will lead to increased intra-cellular calcium, which, in turn will lead to increased insulin resistance. Insulin resistance in type 2 diabetes causes a large amount of insulin to be excreted through the urine.

In Europe, diabetes is referred to as a magnesium wasting disease. Insulin resistance and magnesium loss results in a vicious cycle of worsening insulin resistance and decreasing intra-cellular magnesium.

It is important to remember that a lot of magnesium can be lost through sweating. So, if you exercise and sweat a lot, you will be more prone to suffer from magnesium deficiency.

One key effect of magnesium is that it helps the muscles to relax. Losing magnesium makes the blood vessels constrict, leading to hypertension.

Magnesium has a host of other benefits in the body. It will lower triglycerides, lower LDL, and increase HDL cholesterol.

In a long-term, prospective study, researchers followed 85,060 women and 42,872 men who had no history of diabetes, cardiovascular disease, or cancer at baseline. After 18 years of follow-up in women and 12 years in men, the researchers discovered 4,085 and 1,333 cases of Type 2 diabetes, respectively. In their analysis, the researchers found a significant inverse association between magnesium intake and diabetes risk. In other words, the lower the magnesium intake, the higher the risk of developing diabetes. (14)

In a well-designed clinical study, researchers investigated the relationship between magnesium in the blood and the risk of developing diabetes in 12,128 middle-aged, non-diabetics during a 6 year follow-up. Authors concluded that low magnesium in the blood is a strong indicator of development of Type 2 diabetes among white but not among black individuals. (15)

Excellent sources of Magnesium: Legumes, Nuts, Seeds, Green Leafy Vegetables, Nut Milk

Vanadium

Vanadium is an essential trace mineral that stimulates glucose oxidation and transport. It is also involved in glycogen production in the liver and in muscles. It inhibits the production of glucose from fat and it also inhibits the absorption of glucose from the gut. All of these factors are very important in glucose metabolism.

Several researchers refer to vanadium as the mimicker. This is because vanadium mimics the effect of insulin. It does this by altering the cell membrane function and making the cell membrane insulin receptors more sensitive to insulin.

Vanadium has several other effects on the body. It inhibits cholesterol production, increases the contractibility of the heart muscle, and it even has anti-cancer properties.

Vanadium deficiency will result in slow growth, increased infant mortality, infertility, elevated cholesterol, elevated triglycerides, hypoglycemia, insulin resistance, diabetes, and cardiovascular disease.

In an experimental study in type 2 diabetic mice, researchers found that oral administration of vanadium for 3 weeks decreased blood glucose levels from 236 mg/dl to 143 mg/dl.

In another clinical study, researchers gave vanadium, as vanadyl sulfate, at a dose of 100 mg per day for 3 weeks to six type 2 diabetics. Thesepatientswerealreadybeing treated with diet and sulfonylurea drugs. Their diabetes was quite uncontrolled, with fasting blood glucose of 210 mg/dl and HbA1c of 9.6. After 3 weeks of vanadium, there was a modest improvement in the fasting blood glucose. It came down to 181 mg/dl from 210 mg/dl. More importantly, vanadium decreased insulin resistance at all three levels: liver, muscles, and fat. (16)

In another study, researchers compared the effects of a dose of 100 mg per day of vanadium (as vanadyl sulfate) in moderately obesetype 2 diabeticsversusnon-diabetics. They found that vanadium decreased insulin resistance in the diabetics, but not in the non-diabetics. (17)

The Vitamin D Connection

The Vedda people are out under the tropical sun day after day, soaking up valuable amounts of vitamin D on a continual basis.

Yet, vitamin D deficiency is very common not only in the United States, but throughout the Western world. However, more than 90 percent of Americans are deficient. The ramifications of vitamin D deficiency can be divided into two groups:

- Short-term implications
- Long-term implications

The short-term implications of vitamin D deficiency are muscle aches, fibromyalgia, and depression. However, the long term implications are more serious. There is increased risk for both type 1 and type 2 diabetes. There is also an increased risk for cancer, osteoporosis, and cardiovascular disease.

The main reason that we are experiencing a vitamin D deficiency, even in sunnyclimates, is that we aren't taking enough vitamin D through our diet. Also, we spend way too much time indoors in front of screens and not enough time outside. Then when we do go out, we cover ourselves in sunblock. Smog and pollution also contribute to lack of exposure to Vitamin D.

Another cause of low Vitamin D levels has been the huge popularity of low-fat diets. Over the last half a century, the Western medical community has been pushing the low-fat diet mantra. Vitamin D just happens to be a fat-soluble vitamin, so it will not get into your bloodstream unless there is fat in your food. So, when you are on a low-fat diet, even when you take a supplement to increase your Vitamin D levels, the Vitamin D is not going to be absorbed very well, if at all.

Fortunately, low fat is not the best way to lose weight as we've already discovered. A high soy diet can also cause inhibited Vitamin D deficiency.

Vitamin D is involved with type 1 and type 2 diabetes. Inflammation resistance is involved in the mechanism of type 2 diabetes. This is an inflammation state associated with elevated cytokines levels, which, through oxidative stress, will cause endothelial dysfunction. That means that the lining of the arteries and veins in the body will begin to break down. Lack of vitamin D is a major contributor to this condition.

Increasing your intake of vitamin D will help to defeat type 2 diabetes by decreasing insulin resistance and by defeating endothelial dysfunction.

Obesity is associated with low vitamin D levels. Of course, every obese person is at risk of developing type 2 diabetes. Addressing low vitamin D levels is a vital step in preventing both obesity and type 2 diabetes.

Vitamin D deficiency will actually cause the death of the beta-cells. These are the cells which produce insulin. There are three factors involved in this cell death:

1. Glucose toxicity – high levels of blood glucose
2. Lipotoxicity – elevated cholesterol and triglyceride levels
3. Inflammation

Taking in more vitamin D will preserve the beta cells in the pancreas. These beta cells have awhole lot ofvitamin D receptors. It will also improve insulin release. Low vitamin D levels are known to cause decreased insulin release, though researchers don't know why.

Vitamin D will also reduce the inflammatory damage which can lead to the death of the beta cells.

Scientific evidence now exists to show that proper vitamin D supplementation can prevent type 1 diabetes. One such study comes from Finland. This study began when 10,821 children born in 1966 in northern Finland were enrolled in the study. Frequency of vitamin D supplementation was recorded during the first year of life. At that time, the recommended dose of vitamin D for infants in Finland was 2000 I.U. per day. These children were then followed for 31 years for the development of type 1 diabetes. (18)

Researchers made the amazing discovery: those children who received the daily recommended dose of 2000 I.U. of vitamin D during the first year of their life had an almost 80 percent reduction in the risk for the development of type 1 diabetes compared to those children who received less vitamin D.

This is a ground breaking study! If some drug achieved this kind of results, it would hit the headlines and become the standard of care at once. Sadly, even many diabetes experts are not aware of this astounding study even though it was published in 2001 in the prestigious British medical journal Lancet.

In another excellent study, researchers analyzed a total of 21 prospective studies to explore the relationship between vitamin D deficiency and risk for developing type 2 diabetes. Of the total 76,220 participants, 4,996 individualsdevelopedtype 2 diabetes.

The risk of developing type 2 diabetes was nearly 50 percent less in individuals with the highest levels of vitamin D as compared to the lowest levels. Each 4 ng/ml (equal to 10 nmol/L) increment in vitamin D level was associated with a 4 percent lower risk of developing type 2 diabetes. (19)

Investigators in the US continue to spend millions of dollars in their pursuit of a "drug" to prevent type 1 diabetes. So far, this kind of research has produced disappointing results. Amazingly, they have largely ignored the strong evidence that shows the outstanding role of vitamin D in preventing type 1 diabetes. Vitamin D is not a drug. There is no glory or huge profits in simply telling people to take enough vitamin D.

VIII. VEDDA LIFESTYLE FACTORS

When you compare the Vedda of Sri Lanka and the average person living in the Western world today, their lifestyles could not be more different. It's no secret that our modern lifestyle is bad for our health. So, short of moving to the Sri Lankan jungle, what can be done about it?

We can adopt the principles that underlie the Vedda way of life and adapt them to our situation.

Here are the basic lifestyle principles we can learn from the Vedda.

Movement

The Vedda have an active lifestyle. For the men it revolves around hunting and fishing, while the women are busy cultivating crops and preparing food. They spend very little time sitting around doing nothing.

The message for us: **Exercise**

Healthy Habits

The Vedda do not smoke cigarettes or any form of tobacco. Neither do they abuse their bodies with illegal drugs, alcohol or even with prescription medications.

The message for us:

Quit Smoking and Get off Unnecessary Medications and Recreational Drugs

Lack of Stress

The Vedda live a simple, stress-free life. They don't have to worry about mortgage payments, work deadlines, or traffic jams.

The message for us is: **Learn to De-stress**

Putting the Principles into Action

Exercise

Living the fitness lifestyle is a fantastically rewarding experience. It makes you feel energized, athletic, healthy, and ready for action. But, sometimes, it can be plain hard work. With all of the demands of modern living, slipping into unhealthy habits can often seem like such an easier option. Here are ten key fitness tips to keep you focused on your exercise plan – even when you feel like staying on the couch.

Tip # 1: Carry Your Goal

Your ultimate goal is a healthy body. Break that down to three monthly goals and then write them as if they are already accomplished. An example might be . . .

I have achieved 13 percent body fat and I look awesome.

Write this goal on a card and carry it with you everywhere you go. Read it a minimum of seven times each day.

Tip # 2: Mix It Up

Avoid stagnation by varying your workout routine. Every six weeks, change your program around. Your new program should have an entirely different rep range, set of exercises, and training tempo.

Tip # 3: Train All Day

During commercials, get out of your chair and pump out some push-ups. During the next break, get against the wall for wall squats and, for commercial break three drop down into the plank position. The TV show will be so much more rewarding.

Tip # 4: Eat More Frequently

Eat every three or four waking hours. Doing so will boost your metabolism, help you to better, synthesize protein, and provide you with a constant supply of slow-release carbohydrates to fuel you throughout your day.

Tip # 5: Mix Up Weights and Cardio

Weight training, while focusing on your anaerobic system, also gives your heart and lungs a great workout. Your aerobic system is fully taxed, however when you do work that gets your heart rate to 70 percent of your maximum and keeps it there for twenty minutes.

Tip # 6: HITT It

High Intensity Interval Training is the most effective, time efficient way to get fit and burn fat that we know of. It involves doing repetitive cycles of a cardiovascular movement like cycling, sprinting, or rowing for twenty seconds to your absolute maximum effort and then resting for ten seconds.

Tip # 7: Do a Little When You Feel Like Doing Nothing

Some days even the most motivated of us just don't feel like working out. When that day comes, tell yourself that rather than doing your full workout, you're just going to go to the gym and do ten minutes on the treadmill – no more. Do exactly that and then see how you feel. Chances are, you'll cruise right on into your scheduled workout.

Tip # 8: Take a Week Off

Every six to eight weeks – about the time you switch up your program – take a complete week off from training. This will not only revitalize your workouts (you'll be chomping at the bit to get back to it after a few days), it will also allow your body to recuperate and recover.

Tip # 9: Be Self Aware

Never allow yourself to just go through the motions. When you're exercising, make sure that your mind-muscle connection is plugged in. Feel the working muscle group. Afterwards, monitor the amount of soreness in the worked muscle.

Tip # 10: Hydrate

Water is the number one nutritional intervention that will improve your performance, allowing you to lift heavier weights and recover faster. Drinking water can even give your fat-loss endeavors a boost.

Stop Smoking

Smoking endangers health and life. It has been directly linked to twenty-five life- threatening diseases, including:

- Heart Attack
- Stroke
- Chronic Bronchitis
- Emphysema
- Cancer

There are also social issues that result from smoking. Smokers have foul-smelling breath, discolored teeth and yellowish- brown fingers. Smoking will also cause premature aging.

For diabetics, the dangers of smoking are even greater. Smoking makes it a whole lot harder to balance your blood sugar level and prevent inflammation of your organs. In addition, nicotine has been shown to raise a person's hemoglobin A1-c levels. Hemoglobin A1-c levels are regularly checked in diabetics as an indicator of how well they are controlling blood sugar. Smokers have, on average, Hemoglobin A1-c levels that are one-third higher than non-smokers!

Smoking also leads to elevated blood pressure levels. This makes it harder for your heart and kidneys, which are already working overtime because you are diabetic, to do their jobs. Smoking will also slow down the flow of blood around the body, limiting the amount of oxygen available to organ tissues.

Kicking the Habit

Smoking is a powerful addiction that is understandably hard to break. The best chances of quitting for good come if you can get some help. There are a lot of people and effective therapies that can help you to stop smoking. You may have the inner strength to stop cold turkey or you may prefer to gradually wean yourself off the habit.

Just like riding a bike, giving up smoking usually doesn't happen on the first attempt.

Be prepared to get back on the bike, because it's likely that you will fall off – more than once. Here are some suggestions that have helped others to succeed:

- **Make up your mind to quit:** Become convinced that it is worth the effort. Make a list of all the benefits of quitting.
- **Analyze your smoking behavior:** Record the times and situations that you smoke. This will help you to foresee future situations that may be tempting.
- **Plan a quit date:** Circle it on your calendar. On that day, quit completely.
- **Clear your environment:** Prior to your quit day, get rid of everything associated with smoking, including ashtrays and matches. Clean the tobacco smell from your clothes.
- **Ask others for support:** Publicly share your goal and ask your friends to help and encourage you.
- **Plan to keep busy on quit day:** Exercise and then go to a place that doesn't permit smoking, like a museum or art gallery.
- **Drink plenty of water:** Stay well hydrated. In addition, eat low-calorie foods and snack on celery and carrot sticks.
- **Get rid of nonproductive thinking:** Don't allow yourself to rationalize your situation with thoughts like, "I'll just have one to get me through this stress," or "Smoking is my only vice."
- **Don't fool yourself into thinking that you can be an occasional smoker**
- **Avoid places and situations that will tempt you**
- **Replace the physical act of placing a cigarette in your mouth with sucking on a cinnamon stick**
- **Take up a hobby that keeps your hands busy**
- **Exercise**
- **When you get the urge to smoke, take a shower**

10 Quick & Easy Tips for Lowering Your Stress Level

(1) Exercise

Earlier in this chapter, we talked about the benefits of exercise. Now we're going to go a bit deeper to explore just how important exercise is for stress relief. Exercise is the most underrated and underused antidepressant there is. Studies show that regular cardiovascular exercise greatly improves mental alertness and concentration, reduces stress, and improves overall physical and mental wellbeing. After a mere five minutes of exercise, the body produces endorphins – the happy hormones – that will help bust nervous tension.

(2) Love Yourself with Positive Affirmations

Around 90 percent of our thoughts lie in the subconscious part of the brains. These thoughts include negative feedback that overourlifetimewehavelearned tobe"true" about ourselves. Daily positive affirmations eventually lodge these thoughts into our subconscious and create an overall more positive mind frame. Statements such as "I am good enough" and "I can achieve this" are a great way to start.

(3) Sleep on It

When we start to get stressed, sleep is generally one of the first things to go on the wayside. The body is its own best healer, but it needs sleep to make repairs. When we sleep, the body repairs damaged tissue and recalibrates chemical and hormonal imbalances.

For those who have difficulty getting to sleep, try creating an atmosphere where you feel most at ease. Dim the lights, ensure the room is at a temperature you feel comfortable and leave your electronic devices out of the bedroom – they are not good sleeping partners.

(4) Eat Well

When stressed, it is easy to find ourselves eating all the wrong foods. When facing a looming deadline, the worst thing a stressed person could do is eat out of a takeout box hunched over the computer. Rather, a diet high in fiber and protein with limited carbohydrates is what is needed to sustain us during stressful times.

Contrary to popular opinion, increased coffee intake is not beneficial to dealing with stress and deadlines. In fact, caffeine can wreak havoc on the nervous system.

(5) Set Yourself Up Right for the Coming Day

Taking ten minutes in the evening to organize what you will wear the next day, ensure the kids' school lunches are made, and prepare for the next work day is recommended to reduce any stressors that can start our days off wrong.

Going to sleep knowing that you are preparedforthe comingdayalsoallowsfora more restful slumber without concentrating on the mounting list of things that need to be accomplished the second you wake.

(6) Single Task It

We live in a society with a lot of time pressure. We often envy people who excel at multitasking and cram a ton into their days. But studies have shown that people who chronically multitask experience more anxiety than those who focus on one task at a time.

Many people observe that although they can achieve more in a day through multitasking, they aren't able to do any one thing as well as when they focus on each task individually. Focusing on one task at a time also allows you to feel a sense of accomplishment at each completion point, creating feelings positivity and self-worth.

(7) Music

If music be the food of love, play on. When feeling the effects of stress, music has an amazing ability to drastically shift our mindset, fast. It's easy to find albums of soothing nature sounds. Pick what works best for you and play music that you have a positive connection to.

The next time you are stressed, try removing yourself from a situation for five minutes

to sit or dance. Hearing songs you loved when you were a child has been proven to reduce anxiety by increasing the levels of endorphins your body produces. Try it – it works!

If you're stressed when you're out and about, consider mobile phone and tablet apps that play soothing sounds. They are an excellent way to slow yourself down when you're on the go.

(8) Laugh It Off

It sounds bizarre, but forcing yourself to laugh can actually pull you out of a negative funk. When we laugh, oxygen goes deeper into our lungs, which stimulates the heart and muscles and signals the brain to produce endorphins. Laughter also relaxes tense body muscles. It is next to impossible to have a good giggle with clenched fists – give it a go and feel your body start to relax.

(9) When All Else Fails, Breathe

Our breathing changes when we are feeling anxious. Often our breath becomes short and shallow. It is necessary to increase the length and depth of our breaths to ensure we don't hyperventilate. The best way to do so is to place your hand on your stomach and breathe in through your nose for four seconds. Hold for two seconds and then push as much air as you can for four seconds.

(10) Learn Your Stressors

Learning what stresses you out is a key way of managing anxiety. Take time to figure out what maycauseyou to become anxious and develop coping strategies. For example, does the idea of losing your keys fill you with stress and dread? Get a spare copy made and keep them somewhere safe. Tailor your strategies to what is important to you.

Eliminate Alcohol

Ethyl alcohol (ethanol) is the main ingredient of alcoholic beverages. It is made from the yeast fermentation of starch or sugar. Almost any sweet or starchy food can be turned into alcohol.

Alcohol is not digested by the body. 95 percent of it is absorbed into the bloodstream from the stomach and small intestine within an hour. The other 5 percent is eliminated through the kidneys, lungs, or skin. The liver breaks down, or metabolizes, alcohol. The time it takes to do this depends on whether the alcohol is taken with food. In general, however, it takes three to five hours to completely metabolize 30 ml of alcohol.

In the process of breaking down alcohol, toxic byproducts are released. These toxins are damaging to the liver. They may cause inflammation and lead to the condition known as fatty liver. A person with fatty liver is unable to adequately filter out the dangerous waste products that are coursing around his or her body.

Alcohol consumption diverts your liver from other vital functions. Rather than releasing glucose, it has to clear the toxic waste from your system that comes with the alcohol. This results in lowered glucose production and lowered blood-sugar level.

Excessive alcohol consumption can actually cause liver cells to burst and die. It can also lead to cirrhosis of the liver, which is characterized by irreversible scarring of the liver. Over time this will cause the liver to become lumpy rather than spongy. The scar tissue prevents normal blood flow. This can cause complete liver failure and death. And, because it takes two hours to metabolize a single ounce of alcohol, this damaging effect will continue long after you've consumed your last drop of alcohol.

Alcohol doesn't just cause organ damage to the liver. The pancreas also comes in for a beating. When alcohol is absorbed by the body, it releases a substance called acetaldehyde. This poisonous substance damages the pancreas. One of the jobs that the pancreas does is to contribute to the process of turning food into energy. It secretes enzymes, insulin, and glycogen. Excessive alcohol consumption results in swelling in the pancreas and surrounding blood vessels. This causes the condition known as pancreatitis. Pancreatitis stops the pancreas from working and can lead directly to diabetes. If left unchecked, it can cause death.

Alcohol, of course, doesn't just have a physical effect on your body. Alcohol also impairs your ability to work and go about your daily activities. This is not a good situation for a diabetic. If you are becoming hypoglycemic, your impaired condition may cause you to ignore this dangerous state. Onlookers, too, may simply think that you are drunk and not give you the needed attention.

Alcohol contains calories, and these calories add up very quickly. They are full of carbs, mainly in the form of pure sugar. If taken without food, this can cause low blood glucose by increasing the activity of insulin without food to compensate for it.

The bottom line on alcohol is that it will chip away at all of the good work that you've been doing to gain mastery over your condition. Yet you don't have to let it. You are not a slave to alcohol. Be smart about alcohol by:

- Not having it in the house
- Offering to be the designated driver when you socialize
- When dining out, order tea or mineral water
- Drinking your ten glasses of water per day (you won't want to drink anything else!)

IX. THE FULL BODY DETOX

Take a member of the Vedda community with you to your local supermarket, and he most likely would recognize very few of the thousands of foods in the building. Over the last 100 years, the Western world has done a great job of turning non-food into food. It's been great for the bottom lines of the mega manufacturers of all of these chemically induced foods. But non-food has been negatively affecting the health of millions of people. And the main vehicle that has been fast tracking all of those people to an early grave is diabetes.

In order to benefit from the life-giving benefits of a Vedda-inspired eating plan, you've first got to rid yourbodyof the myriad level of toxins that have accumulated.

That means undertaking a one-day detox.

Acid Overload

One of the most serious impacts of the infestation of toxins into our bodies is that it has played havoc with our pH levels. The balance between an acidic and an alkaline liquid internal environment is the key determinant of our overall well-being. The body functions optimally at a slightly alkaline state (pH level of 7.4). When the fluid within our bodies becomes too acidic, we compensate by leeching minerals from our organs, muscles, ligaments and bones. This leaves those involuntary donor body parts susceptible to illness.

In order to correct our pH balance toward that magic number of 7.4, we need to remove acid from our systems. That means getting rid of the harmful toxins that we have ingested, either through our foods or through the atmosphere.

Why Detox?

Your body is constantly working. Even when you're not eating it's digesting the food from a previous meal. That doesn't leave much time for detoxing. It's a bit like a commercial kitchen that's going twenty-four hours a day. Employees are so busy cooking that they never get a chance to clean the oven or mop the floor. It's only when they shut down production that they can clean the place up. A detox allows you to clean out your internal oven.

The main goal of detoxing is to eliminate toxins from your body. This will improve your energy, give your liver and digestive system a break, clear up your skin, improve your health, and help you to lose weight. It puts your body in a position where it can build, defend, and restore itself.

Just What is a Detox?

The word detox actually means to cleanse the blood. This is done by removing impurities from the liver. That is where the toxins that we ingest are processed for elimination. Other areas of the body that detoxify include the blood, the skin, the kidneys, the lymphatic system, and the lungs. However, these natural detoxification centers can easily get clogged up, preventing them from working properly. Detoxification is the process by which we clean up the internal house that we live in.

Keep in mind that a detox doesn't mean fasting. Although a detox may involve a period of fasting, it is more about introducing foods that will assist you to flush out the toxins while giving your body a rest from your normal eating pattern.

Time to Detox

Those nasty toxins have been hijacking your body for way too long. Now that you're aware of it, it's time to do something about it. There are a whole host of detox regimens that you can followandyou should definitely do your own research to find one that suits your specific requirements.

If you are new to detoxing, you may choose to begin with a one-day cleanse. This will give your body a chance to take a break from all of the pressure that it is under to make sense of the unnatural foods that it is being forced to cope with. This is a great opportunity to dip your toe into the detoxing waters. It will be like giving your body a whole-day tune up. You'll need a juicer so that you can make soups and juices.

What to Remove

The first things to eliminate from your diet are alcohol and coffee. Next cut out all fast foods, junk foods, and fried foods. Then get rid of all processed foods and grains. After that get rid of all meat and dairy foods.

What to Add

Replace the toxin-laden gunk foods with foods that will cleanse and reinvigorate your body. Here are seven great choices . . .

- 3 organically grown fruits
- 3 leafy green vegetables
- 3 legumes
- 3 Natural raw seeds

Finally, here are ten tips to make your one- day detox a big success:

- Select foods close to nature
- Start the day with a piece of fruit or lemon juice in hot water
- Include fresh fruits and salads
- Include fresh vegetables
- Include hormone-free, free-range, organic protein
- Use celtic salt
- Drink herbal teas
- Choose cold-pressed olive oil or unrefined coconut oil
- Apple cider vinegar can be used for digestive stimulation
- Include nuts and seeds (activated is best)

I know someone who lost her one-carat diamond while mowing the lawn. The stone, which had been in her family for generations, fell out of its setting because the prongs were loose. If she had brought her ring in regularly for cleaning, she could have kept it in good condition. Our bodies are the same. In fact, our bodies are the most priceless things we have. Give your body the respect it deserves by cleaning it out every now and then. Once you've tried a cleanse once, you'll be amazed at how much more alive you feel. Try it for yourself.

YOUR 30-DAY BLOOD SUGAR BUSTING PROTOCOL

During the course of this book, you have learned a ton of information about the lifestyle of a remote Sri Lankan culture and how it can help you to defeat diabetes. In this chapter, we will review each of these vital steps

To cure diabetes the Vedda way, you absolutely must

- Undertake a daily detox
- Drink ten 8-ounce glasses of water every day
- Get at least eight hours of sleep every night
- Schedule personal, relaxed hobby time each week
- Get rid of nonproductive thought patterns
- Do a minimum of twenty minutes of exercise five times per week
- Nix Sugar – use only healthy substitutes like honey, stevia, fruits, and spices
- Remove grains, preservatives, and MSG
- Eat plenty of protein, relying on poultry, lamb, fish and plant proteins
- Eat whole, fresh foods
- Eat coconut daily
- Do not consume fruit or vegetable juices
- Do not consume canned foods
- Supplement with Vitamin D – 800 IU
- daily
- Supplement with Magnesium – 400mg daily
- Supplement with Chromium – 1000 mcg daily
- Consume ginger root daily

To cure diabetes in thirty days, you MUST remove the following from your life:

- Sugar
- Alcohol
- Tobacco
- Artificial sweeteners
- Stress
- MSG
- White flour, pasta and rice
- Instant and processed foods
- Canned foods
- Fruit and vegetable juices

There it is – over the next thirty days, you WILL be on your way to defeating diabetes if you implement each of the bullet points in our 30-Day Blood Sugar Busting Protocol. In the process you will have changed your lifestyle to include more exercise and less stress, modeling the ways of the Vedda to the greatest extent possible.

You will do all of those without the use of medications. There'll be no injections and no hanging around in waiting rooms. The diabetes-defeating wisdom of the Vedda has freed you from all of that.

Your 30-Day Beat Diabetes Shopping List

BUY THIS...	FOR THIS...
Limes	Detox
Cider Apple Vinegar	Detox
Pure Honey	Detox
Turmeric	Detox
Cayenne Pepper	Detox
Rosemary	Detox
Lemons	Lunch
Poultry	Lunch
Lamb	Lunch
Fish	Lunch, Dinner
Eggs	Breakfast, Lunch, Dinner
Beans	Lunch, Dinner
Romaine Lettuce	Breakfast, Lunch, Dinner
Carrots	Breakfast, Lunch, Dinner
Cucumbers	Breakfast, Lunch, Dinner
Peppers	Breakfast, Lunch, Dinner
Onions	Breakfast, Lunch, Dinner

Spinach	Breakfast, Lunch, Dinner
Coconut	Breakfast, Lunch, Dinner
Tomatoes	Breakfast, Lunch, Dinner
Asparagus	Breakfast, Lunch, Dinner
Broccoli	Breakfast, Lunch, Dinner
Apples	Snack
Peaches	Snack
Plums	Snack
Salmon	Lunch, Dinner
Canary Seeds	Lunch, Dinner
Nuts	Breakfast, Lunch, Dinner
Garlic	Breakfast, Lunch, Dinner
Zucchini	Breakfast, Lunch, Dinner
Vitamin D Supps	Supplement
Magnesium Supps	Supplement
Ginseng	Supplement
Zinc Supps	Supplement
Pycnogenol	Supplement
Vanadium	Supplement

Your Daily Meal Schedule

While your daily food choices will vary according to your individual preferences, here is a daily template which can serve as a guide to the types of foods you should be eating at each meal.

Meal	What to Eat
Breakfast	Salad, Shake, 1 Egg, Vegetables
Brunch	Fruit
Lunch	Salmon, Poultry, Lamb, Peas, Vegetables
Afternoon	Snack Fruit
Dinner	Salmon, Fish, Poultry, Peas, Vegetables

The 30-Day Protocol

(All Recipes in Following Section)

Day	What to Eat	What Supps to Take	What to Do
Day 1	One-Day Detox: • 1 Tablespoon lime juice • 1 Tablespoon apple cider vinegar • 1 Tablespoon pure honey • 1/8 Teaspoon turmeric • 1/8 Teaspoon cayenne pepper • 1/8 teaspoon rosemary Fresh Fruit		ONE-DAY DETOX Drink ten 8-ounce glasses water
Day 2	Breakfast: 2 HARDBOILED EGGS/ COCONUT MILK/BANANA Lunch: MUSHROOM AND DRY FRUIT PILAF Dinner: CHICKEN AND MUSHROOM STEW	• Vitamin D - 800 IU • Magnesium - 400mg • Chromium - 1000 mcg	Eliminate ALL sugary, carb laden junk food from your home! Exercise twenty mins Drink ten 8-ounce glasses water

Day 3	Breakfast: MUSHROOM OMELETTE Lunch: VEGETABLE SOUP Dinner: PORK STEW WITH APPLE CIDER VINEGAR	• Vitamin D - 800 IU • Magnesium - 400mg • Chromium - 1000 mcg	Eliminate ALL sugary, carb laden junk food from your diet! **Exercise twenty mins** Drink ten 8-ounce glasses water
Day 4	Breakfast: ITALIAN SAUSAGE WITH BLACK BEANS Lunch: CHICKEN WINGS IN PEANUT BUTTER Dinner: CRANBERRY MEATBALLS	• Vitamin D - 800 IU • Magnesium - 400mg • Chromium - 1000 mcg	Eliminate ALL sugary, carb laden junk food from your diet! **Exercise twenty mins**
Day 5	Breakfast: PALEO BREAD Lunch: TANGY BARBEQUE SAUSAGES Dinner: STUFFED CABBAGE ROLLE LEAFS	• Vitamin D - 800 IU • Magnesium - 400mg • Chromium - 1000 mcg	Eliminate ALL sugary, carb laden junk food from your diet! **Exercise twenty mins** Drink ten 8-ounce glasses water

Vedda Blood Sugar Remedy

Day	Meals	Supplements	Activity
Day 6	Breakfast: ALMOND FLOUR COCONUT WAFFLES Lunch: PORK WRAPS WITH HONEY Dinner: SWEET AND SOUR PORK	• Vitamin D - 800 IU • Magnesium - 400mg • Chromium - 1000 mcg	Hobby Time
Day 7	Breakfast: POACHED EGGS IN AVOCADO Lunch: SALMON & TUNA MUFFINS WITH LIME DIPPING SAUCE Dinner: PIQUANT CHICKEN	• Vitamin D - 800 IU • Magnesium - 400mg • Chromium - 1000 mcg	Hobby Time
Day 8	Breakfast: VEGETABLE SOUP Lunch: TANGY BARBEQUE SAUSAGES Dinner: BARBECUE TURKEY WRAPS	• Vitamin D - 800 IU • Magnesium - 400mg • Chromium - 1000 mcg	Exercise twenty mins Drink ten 8-ounce glasses water

Day 9	Breakfast: COCONUT CHIPS, ALMONDS, AND FRUIT Lunch: BEEF AND VEGETABLE SOUP Dinner: CRANBERRY MEATBALLS	• Vitamin D - 800 IU • Magnesium - 400mg • Chromium - 1000 mcg	Exercise twenty mins Drink ten 8-ounce glasses water
Day 10	Breakfast: MAYONNAISE FREE DEVILLED EGGS Lunch: GARLIC SHRIMP IN COCONUT MILK Dinner: CRANBERRY MEATBALLS	• Vitamin D - 800 IU • Magnesium - 400mg • Chromium - 1000 mcg	Exercise twenty mins Drink ten 8-ounce glasses water
Day 11	Breakfast: ITALIAN SAUSAGE WITH BLACK BEANS Lunch: CHICKEN WINGS IN PEANUT BUTTER Dinner: CRANBERRY MEATBALLS	• Vitamin D - 800 IU • Magnesium - 400mg • Chromium - 1000 mcg	Exercise twenty mins Drink ten 8-ounce glasses water

Day 12	Breakfast: PALEO BREAD Lunch: TANGY BARBEQUE SAUSAGES Dinner: STUFFED CABBAGE ROLLED LEAVES	• Vitamin D - 800 IU • Magnesium - 400mg • Chromium - 1000 mcg	Exercise twenty mins Drink ten 8-ounce glasses water
Day 13	Breakfast: ALMOND FLOUR COCONUT WAFFLES Lunch: PORK WRAPS WITH HONEY Dinner: SWEET AND SOUR PORK	• Vitamin D - 800 IU • Magnesium - 400mg • Chromium - 1000 mcg	Exercise twenty mins Drink ten 8-ounce glasses water
Day 14	Breakfast: POACHED EGGS IN AVOCADO Lunch: SALMON & TUNA MUFFINS WITH LIME DIPPING SAUCE Dinner: PIQUANT CHICKEN	• Vitamin D - 800 IU • Magnesium - 400mg • Chromium - 1000 mcg	Hobby Time Drink ten 8-ounce glasses water

Day 15	Breakfast: VEGETABLE SOUP Lunch: TANGY BARBEQUE SAUSAGES Dinner: BARBECUE TURKEY WRAPS	• Vitamin D - 800 IU • Magnesium - 400mg • Chromium - 1000 mcg	**Hobby Time** Drink ten 8-ounce glasses water
Day 16	Breakfast: MAYONNAISE FREE DEVILLED EGGS Lunch: GARLIC SHRIMP IN COCONUT MILK Dinner: CRANBERRY MEATBALLS	• Vitamin D - 800 IU • Magnesium - 400mg • Chromium - 1000 mcg	**Exercise twenty mins** Drink ten 8-ounce glasses water
Day 17	Breakfast: MUSHROOM OMELETTE Lunch: VEGETABLE SOUP Dinner: PORK STEW WITH APPLE CIDER VINEGAR	• Vitamin D - 800 IU • Magnesium - 400mg • Chromium - 1000 mcg	**Exercise twenty mins** Drink ten 8-ounce glasses water

Day	Meals	Supplements	Activity
Day 18	Breakfast: ITALIAN SAUSAGE WITH BLACK BEANS Lunch: CHICKEN WINGS IN PEANUT BUTTER Dinner: CRANBERRY MEATBALLS	• Vitamin D - 800 IU • Magnesium - 400mg • Chromium - 1000 mcg	Exercise twenty mins
Day 19	Breakfast: WALNUTS AND RAISINS WITH COCONUT FLAKES Lunch: TANGY BARBEQUE SAUSAGES Dinner: STUFFED CABBAGE ROLLE LEAFS	• Vitamin D - 800 IU • Magnesium - 400mg • Chromium - 1000 mcg	Exercise twenty mins Drink ten 8-ounce glasses water
Day 20	Breakfast: ALMOND FLOUR COCONUT WAFFLES Lunch: PORK WRAPS WITH HONEY Dinner: SWEET AND SOUR PORK	• Vitamin D - 800 IU • Magnesium - 400mg • Chromium - 1000 mcg	Exercise twenty mins Drink ten 8-ounce glasses water

Day 21

Breakfast:
POACHED EGGS IN AVOCADO

Lunch:
SALMON & TUNA MUFFINS WITH LIME DIPPING SAUCE

Dinner:
PIQUANT CHICKEN

- Vitamin D - 800 IU
- Magnesium - 400mg
- Chromium - 1000 mcg

Hobby Time

Drink ten 8-ounce glasses water

Day 22

Breakfast:
VEGETABLE SOUP

Lunch:
TANGY BARBEQUE SAUSAGES

Dinner:
BARBECUE TURKEY WRAPS

- Vitamin D - 800 IU
- Magnesium - 400mg
- Chromium - 1000 mcg

Hobby Time

Drink ten 8-ounce glasses water

Day 23

Breakfast:
MAYONNAISE FREE DEVILLED EGGS

Lunch:
GARLIC SHRIMP IN COCONUT MILK

Dinner:
CRANBERRY MEATBALLS

- Vitamin D - 800 IU
- Magnesium - 400mg
- Chromium - 1000 mcg

Exercise twenty mins

Drink ten 8-ounce glasses water

Day 24	Breakfast: MUSHROOM OMELETTE Lunch: VEGETABLE SOUP Dinner: PORK STEW WITH APPLE CIDER VINEGAR	• Vitamin D - 800 IU • Magnesium - 400mg • Chromium - 1000 mcg	Exercise twenty mins Drink ten 8-ounce glasses water
Day 25	Breakfast: ITALIAN SAUSAGE WITH BLACK BEANS Lunch: CHICKEN WINGS IN PEANUT BUTTER Dinner: CRANBERRY MEATBALLS	• Vitamin D - 800 IU • Magnesium - 400mg • Chromium - 1000 mcg	Exercise twenty mins
Day 26	Breakfast: WALNUTS AND RAISINS WITH COCONUT FLAKES Lunch: TANGY BARBEQUE SAUSAGES Dinner: STUFFED CABBAGE ROLLE	• Vitamin D - 800 IU • Magnesium - 400mg • Chromium - 1000 mcg	Exercise twenty mins Drink ten 8-ounce glasses water

Day 27	Breakfast: ALMOND FLOUR COCONUT WAFFLES Lunch: PORK WRAPS WITH HONEY Dinner: SWEET AND SOUR PORK	• Vitamin D - 800 IU • Magnesium - 400mg • Chromium - 1000 mcg	**Exercise twenty mins** Drink ten 8-ounce glasses water
Day 28	Breakfast: POACHED EGGS IN AVOCADO Lunch: SALMON & TUNA MUFFINS WITH LIME DIPPING SAUCE Dinner: PIQUANT CHICKEN	• Vitamin D - 800 IU • Magnesium - 400mg • Chromium - 1000 mcg	**Exercise twenty mins** Drink ten 8-ounce glasses water
Day 29	Breakfast: VEGETABLE SOUP Lunch: TANGY BARBEQUE SAUSAGES Dinner: BARBECUE TURKEY WRAPS	• Vitamin D - 800 IU • Magnesium - 400mg • Chromium - 1000 mcg	**Exercise twenty mins** Drink ten 8-ounce glasses water

| Day 30 | Breakfast:
MAYONNAISE FREE DEVILLED EGGS

Lunch:
GARLIC SHRIMP IN COCONUT MILK

Dinner:
CRANBERRY MEATBALLS | • Vitamin D - 800 IU
• Magnesium - 400mg
• Chromium - 1000 mcg | **Exercise twenty mins**

Drink ten 8-ounce glasses water |

The Recipes

BREAKFAST

It is really important that you eat a real, healthy breakfast. The heartier the first meal of the day is, the better. A decent breakfast will allow you to fire up your metabolism and get your hunger under control for the coming day.

Want to know how important eating breakfast is? A landmark study by the US National Weight Control Registry (NWCR) identified that, of members who had lost an average of sixty-six pounds and kept it off for five years, 90 percent of them ate breakfast on most days of the week. Breakfast eaters also reported higher levels of physical activity. In contrast, breakfast skippers tended to make poor food choices. Don't be one of them; make it your routine every day to have a nutritious breakfast so that you're well fueled and mentally sharp for the day ahead.

MUSHROOM OMELETTE

Serves: 1

Ingredients

- 1 cup mushrooms, chopped 2 teaspoons nondairy milk 1/2 cup egg beaters
- 1 teaspoon olive oil 1 dash pepper
- 1 dash salt

Preparation

- Stir fry mushroom in olive oil for four minutes or until soft.
- Combine egg substitute with milk, salt, and pepper and oil skillet with olive oil.
- Heat skillet for thirty seconds and add egg mixture to it.
- Cook for two minutes to set; add in mushrooms cook for two more minutes.
- When omelet is almost done, turn over to flat plate and use a spatula to put it back to pan to cook the other side.
- Serve warm with veggies of choice.

ITALIAN SAUSAGE WITH BLACK BEANS

Serves: 3

Ingredients

- 12 oz Italian sausage, chopped
- ½ a medium-sized onion, chopped
- ½ cup canned black beans
- ½ cup salsa
- ½ cup tomato puree
- 1 ½ green chilies, minced 2-3 basil leaves
- teaspoon pepper
- ¾ tablespoon salt
- 1 teaspoon vegetable oil

Preparation

1. Sauté the onions and chilies for about 5-6 minutes in a crockpot with olive oil.

2. Add remaining ingredients, cover the lid, and cook for three to four hours on slow heat.

MAYONNAISE FREE DEVILLED EGGS

Serves: 4

Ingredients

- 6 large hard-boiled eggs 1/4 cup pureed avocado 1 dash black pepper
- 2 teaspoons vinegar
- 1 dash salt

Preparation

- Peel eggs and cut into half lengthwise.
- Remove yolks and keep aside.
- Combine yolks with other ingredients and mix until smooth.
- Spoon equal amount of yolk mixture into egg white halves and serve.

WALNUT RAISINS WITH COCONUT FLAKES

Serves: 1

Ingredients

- 1/4 cup walnuts
- 1/4 cup raisins
- 1/2 cup unsweetened coconut flakes or chips

Preparation

- Mix all ingredients together in a bowl.
- Serve plain or with nondairy milk.

ALMOND FLOUR COCONUT WAFFLES

Serves: 1-2

Ingredients

- 1 ½ cups almond flour/meal 2 eggs, whisked
- ¼ cup canned coconut milk
- ¼ cup unsweetened shredded coconut
- 1 tablespoon arrowroot powder or coconut flour 1 tablespoon raw honey
- 1 teaspoon vanilla extract
- ½ teaspoon baking soda
- ½ teaspoon sea salt
- ½ teaspoon cinnamon

Preparation

- Whisk eggs in a medium-large sized bowl.
- Add coconut milk and whisk together with eggs.
- Next mix in almond flour, shredded coconut, arrowroot powder, and baking soda.
- Lastly, add in honey, vanilla, salt, and cinnamon. Mix together thoroughly.
- Pour into waffle iron and heat until cooked through.

POACHED EGGS IN AVOCADO

Serves: 2

Ingredients

- 3 Eggs
- 3 Avocados, halved with pits removed

Preparation

- Poach eggs according to your taste and place them in avocadoes, in the bowl where the pits were.
- Sprinkle with pepper.

VEGETABLE SOUP

Serves: 2

Ingredients

- Green Beans Celery Zucchini Yellow Squash Red Peppers Leeks
- Onions Garlic
- Shredded Cabbage Vegetable Broth Oregano
- Basil Salt

Preparation

- Cut up and combine vegetables in a pot of heated vegetable broth.
- Bring to the boil and then simmer for fifteen minutes.
- Add salt, oregano, and basil for flavor.

LUNCH

Lunch can be a tricky meal. Often we're not at home when we eat it. But, whether you're eating at home, the office, or on the go, what you put in your mouth at midday can either keep your metabolism humming or send you spiraling toward mid-afternoon cravings. Here are five key tips to allow you to make smart lunch choices:

(1) Pack in protein

(2) Use dark greens as a salad base

(3) Add color to your salads

(4) Fill up on fiber

(5) Go with smoothies (add frozen fruit)

CHICKEN WINGS IN PEANUT BUTTER

Serves: 2

Ingredients

- 5-6 chicken wings
- 3 tablespoons peanut butter 1 teaspoon salt
- 1 tablespoon ground ginger 1 cup water

Preparation

1. Combine all the ingredients in a slow cooker and cover.

2. Slow cook this dish for five to six hours (initial three hours on

slow heat, the next two hours on medium heat).

Serving

Serve it hot and top with roasted almonds.

Variation

Try using pork instead of chicken.

MUSHROOM AND DRY FRUIT PILAF

Serves: 2 or 3

Ingredients

- ½ cup sliced button mushrooms 2 cups chopped almonds
- 1 cup chopped cashews 2 cloves of cardamom
- 1 chopped onion
- 2 minced garlic cloves 1 teaspoon salt
- 1 teaspoon olive oil 1 cup water

Preparation

1. Sauté garlic cloves and onion in a slow cooker until they turn slightly brown.

2. Add remaining ingredients and cook for about 6-7 hours. Serve hot.

Variation

Instead of mushrooms, you can also use chicken pieces.

TANGY BARBEQUE SAUSAGES

Serves: 3

Ingredients

- 1 large onion, chopped 12 oz smoked sausages
- 2 tablespoons apple cider vinegar
- ½ cup tomato puree
- 1 teaspoon paprika powder 1 teaspoon salt
- teaspoon cayenne pepper
- ½ cup water
- 1 teaspoon olive oil

Preparation

1. Sauté the onion in a slow cooker.

2. Add remaining ingredients, cover and cook for 4-5 hours

PORK WRAPS WITH HONEY

Serves: 3

Ingredients

- 12 oz boneless pork, trimmed and shredded 1 roughly chopped onion
- ½ cup water
- 2 tablespoons Worcestershire sauce
- ¼ cup tomato puree
- 1 teaspoon ginger garlic paste 2 tablespoons honey
- 1 teaspoon salt Romaine lettuce leaves

Preparation

1. Add all the ingredients except lettuce in a slow cooker.
2. Cook this filling for 11-12 hours.

Serve filling wrapped in lettuce leaves.

Variation

Try with chicken instead of pork.

GARLIC SHRIMP IN COCONUT MILK

Serves: 2

Ingredients

- 12 oz peeled shrimp 1 tablespoon olive oil 4 minced garlic cloves
- ¾ cup coconut milk Coriander leaves
- 1 teaspoon lemon juice 1 teaspoon salt

Preparation

1. Sauté minced garlic with olive oil in a slow cooker.//
2. Add remaining ingredients and cook for five hours on slow heat.

EASY GUACAMOLE SALAD

Serves: 3-4

Ingredients

- 3 small avocados, chopped
- large ripe but firm tomato, chopped 1 small green chili, chopped
- 1 can black beans
- ½ small onion, chopped
- ½ tsp freshly grated lime zest
- ½ cup coriander, chopped
- tablespoons of lemon or lime juice 3 tablespoons olive oil, cold pressed 1 pinch of Celtic sea salt
- ¼ tsp ground cayenne pepper
- ½ tsp minced garlic

Preparation

- Place the tomato, green chili, black beans, onion, coriander, and lime zest into a large bowl.
- Whisk together the lime juice, olive oil, sea salt, garlic, and cayenne pepper. Pour over the vegetables and toss well.
- Just before serving, fold the avocado into the salad. Serve at room temperature.

SALMON & TUNA MUFFINS WITH LIME DIPPING SAUCE

Serves: 2-3

Ingredients

- 3 cloves garlic, crushed 2 teaspoons sesame oil
- teaspoon chopped lemongrass 1 tablespoon chopped ginger
- 1 egg, beaten
- tablespoons chopped coriander 16 oz canned tuna or salmon
- 1 teaspoon red chili (optional)
- Dipping Sauce: ½ cup rice wine vinegar, 2 tablespoons lime juice, 1 large red chili, 1 tablespoon coriander
- Preheat oven to 350 F. Line mini muffin tray.

Preparation

- Place all ingredients (except ingredients for dipping sauce) into food processor until well combined.
- Spoon mixture into muffin tin and bake for ten minutes or until cooked through.
- To make dipping sauce, place all ingredients into a bowl and mix well.
- Serve with a nice salad.

DINNER

In the Western world we don't do dinner very well. We generally eat way too much, and not enough of the right stuff. In fact, a survey revealed that the healthfulness of what we eat decreases 1.7 percent for every hour that passes in the day. Other research reports that dinner is 15.9 percent less healthy than breakfast on average. This section gives you the power to maintain your healthy lifestyle until your head hits the pillow.

CHICKEN AND MUSHROOM STEW

Serves: 2

Ingredients

- 1 lb chopped chicken breasts
- ½ cup button mushrooms 1 teaspoon oregano
- 2 celery stalks, sliced 1 teaspoon salt
- ¼ cup red wine
- 2 minced garlic cloves
- ½ cup tomato puree

Preparation

1. Combine all the ingredients in a slow cooker and cover.
2. Cook for six hours.

Variation

Add vegetables like cabbage or carrots.

PORK STEW WITH APPLE CIDER VINEGAR

Serves: 2

Ingredients

- 1 lb chopped pork roast
- 2 tablespoons apple cider vinegar
- ½ cup chopped sweet potato 1 teaspoon thyme
- 1 teaspoon parsley
- 1 teaspoon salt
- 1 cup water

Preparation

1. Combine all ingredients, mix well and transfer it to a slow cooker.

2. Cover and cook for ten to eleven hours.

STUFFED CABBAGE ROLLED LEAVES

Serves: 3

Ingredients

- 5-6 cabbage leaves
- ¾ lb sliced turkey
- 2 minced garlic cloves 2 chopped onions
- 1 small apple, chopped 1 teaspoon salt
- 1 teaspoon paprika powder
- teaspoon Worcestershire sauce

Preparation

1. Mix the turkey, garlic, onions, apple, paprika, salt, and Worcestershire sauce in a bowl.

2. Place filling into cabbage leaves, fold leaves and secure each with a toothpick.

3. Cook wraps on slow heat for seven to eight hours in a crockpot.

Serving

Serve with Worcestershire sauce.

Variation

Try adding Zucchini or broccoli to the filling.

SWEET AND SOUR PORK

Serves: 6

Ingredients

- 4-5 pork chops
- 1 ½ cups diced carrots 1 ½ cups broccoli florets
- 10 oz chopped pineapple (canned) 1 chopped green bell pepper
- ½ teaspoon minced garlic cloves
- ½ teaspoon minced ginger
- 2 ½ tablespoons Worcestershire sauce 2 tablespoons vinegar
- ½ teaspoons salt

Preparation

1. Add all the ingredients except pineapple to a crockpot and cover.

2. Let the dish cook for 7-8 hours. Add pineapple and cover. Let sit for 30 minutes before serving.

PIQUANT CHICKEN

Serves: 3

Ingredients

- 1 lb chopped chicken 1 finely chopped onion 2 minced garlic cloves
- 1 ½ tablespoon curry powder   1 teaspoon apple cider vinegar 6-7 raisins
- 5-6 almonds
- ½ cup tomato puree

Preparation

1. In a slow cooker, sauté the onions and bell peppers.

2. Add remaining ingredients and cook for seven hours.

BARBECUE TURKEY WRAPS

Serves: 3 or 4

Ingredients

- 1 lb minced turkey
- 1 ½ cups finely chopped tomatoes
- ½ cup tomato puree 1 finely chopped onion 3 minced garlic cloves
- 1 tablespoon Worcestershire sauce 2 tablespoons barbecue sauce
- 1 teaspoon salt
- 1 teaspoon paprika powder 1 teaspoon olive oil Romaine lettuce

Preparation

1. In a slow cooker, sauté the garlic and the onion until slightly browned.

2. Add remaining ingredients except lettuce, cover and let cook for three hours.

3. Fill the mixture in the lettuce leaves and secure with a toothpick.

CRANBERRY MEATBALLS

Serves: 3

Ingredients

- 1 lb ground beef
- 1 cup cranberries, dried
- ½ cup cranberry puree
- 5 tablespoons orange juice 2 tablespoons lemon juice 1 ½ teaspoon salt
- teaspoon pepper
- 1 teaspoon cumin powder 2 tablespoons honey
- eggs, beaten
- teaspoons olive oil

Preparation

- Mix ground beef with cranberries, salt, pepper, and cumin powder and shape into small meatballs.
- Sauté in olive oil in slow cooker until meatballs are slightly browned. Add remaining ingredients, cover and cook for 3-4 hours on slow heat.

Serving

Serve them in a bowl with some parsley and a slice of lime on top.

Variation

Cranberries can be easily substituted with strawberries or even blueberries.

X. YOUR DIABETES - FREE FUTURE

Becoming diabetes free is like being unshackled from a huge weight. You've been dragging this label around for a long time – and it's become a part of who you are.

With the application of the Vedda-based wisdom that has formed the basis of this book, you will be forever free of those shackles. Diabetes will be a part of your past – the person who you used to be, but no longer. That means . . .

- **NO MORE** finger pricks or test strips.
- **NO MORE** injections.
- **NO MORE** having to deny yourself the foods you love.
- **NO MORE** having to live your life with the constant worry of crashing hanging over you, or ending up in a diabetic coma.
- And **NO MORE** fear of having your life cut drastically short, devastating the lives of those you love.

You've got your health back and now you're ready to start living.

Make the most of every day!

Made in the USA
Lexington, KY
13 October 2017